Protect Yourself!

HOW TO STAY SAFE
IN AN UNSAFE
WORLD

Protect Yourself!

HOW TO STAY SAFE IN AN UNSAFE WORLD

RON DANIELS

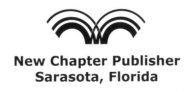

New Chapter Publisher
Sarasota, Florida

Protect Yourself!
How to Stay Safe in an Unsafe World

Published by New Chapter Publisher

ISBN 978-0-982-7918-8-2

New Chapter Publisher
32 South Osprey Ave.
Suite 102
Sarasota, FL 34236
tel. 941-954-4690
www.newchapterpublisher.com

Protect Yourself! How to Stay Safe in an Unsafe World
is distributed by Midpoint Trade Books

Printed in the United States of America

Cover design and layout:
Shaw Creative, www.shawcreativegroup.com

Dedication

To my wife, Sheila,
who lovingly shares with me
all of the big and little challenges of life
and gives me confidence in the future.

And to my children,
Joshua, Jeremy, Jonathan and Priscilla,
who make my life complete.

Contents

ACKNOWLEDGMENTS

There are numerous people who helped and supported me during the time I worked on this book, and I want to thank as many of them as I can remember.

Words cannot express the gratitude and love I feel for my mother and dad, Sylvia and John Daniels, my grandmother, Maggie, and my deceased grandfather, who all taught me important values to live by. I am fortunate to have a wonderful family: my wife, Sheila, and my children Joshua, Jeremy, Jonathan and Priscilla—Jeremy, thank you for helping with the cover of this book. I am also grateful to my in-laws, Franco and Mara, for their love. I appreciate my brothers and sisters for the significant roles they've played in my life. And I want to give a special thanks to my extended family of children, Courtney, Austin and little Joey, and their lovely grandmother, Angela and stepgrandfather, Ron Rutherford, who helped me with statistical research.

Many law enforcement officers have been an inspiration to me, notably former sheriff deputy for the Aero Squad, Ron Browne and his wife, Celia. I'd also like to thank Constable Victor Trevino, his wife, Sylvia, and their family (thank you, Victor, for giving me the time to focus on writing this book), Chief Lopez, Captain Barry, B.J. Yoder and Jarrel Caldwell. I am grateful to my former superiors who have become good friends. They include Chief C.O. Bradford, Chief Michael Tippitt and his wife and family, and Constable Ruben Davis and his wife.

Willie Greason, formerly of the U.S. Marshals Service, has been a model of courage and contagious enthusiasm. Bobby Gillham, former FBI special agent in charge, and his wife, Bobby, have provided wisdom and guidance. Ron Foster provided military expertise and opened doors. at Fort Hood. And I have been honored to have former Houston mayor and U.S drug czar, Lee P. Brown, as a mentor who has been unstinting with his time and support.

Thanks to Assistant District Attorney Mark Herman, his wife, Barb, and their family, who have taught me much about staying true to my dreams; and to Rick and Laura Cayton for making me realize that the glass is always half full, and for introducing me to J.T. Bowyer and his family, who have become an intricate part of my life. Thanks also to Mark and Pam Zastrow, who have shared my dedication to my mission to help others achieve safety; to Dan, Angela and McKenzie Clarke, whose values and faith have been an inspiration; and to Rudy Tomjanovich, a great basketball coach, for understanding why I dedicated my life to law enforcement.

I want to give a special thanks to Joey Kaczmarek and his wife Ruth—Joey, you are a great business partner and friend—and to Steven James and his wife Erica and their family—Steve, I'm proud to have you on my staff.

I am deeply grateful to my editor, Chris Angermann, for working side by side with me on this book and becoming a good friend. I also want to thank Ivana Lucic, president of New Chapter Publisher, for believing in my manuscript, and to acknowledge Tom Madden and Kim Morgan of TransMedia for first recognizing its value and potential.

Thanks to the people who have helped me on the pathway to success. They are Jody and Mike Binkley, Whitney Acke, Rob Fee, Booker Loud, Cecilia and Richard Keiser, Rolando Martinez, Jose and Winnie Zombrano, their children Pamela and Jose Jr. and their nephew Flavio, and especially John Denton, R.J.M and Bernard Pink, whose friendship and encouragement I truly appreciate.

Thanks also to the many good friends who have supported me throughout the writing of this book, including Trevor and Herminia Bello and their children Chris, Trevor and Cody; Michael Carter, Jackie Duyka Shaun, and Jamie Kelly and their wonderful families; Robert Barr, AJ Rios, Danny Vela, James Russell, Ishmael Johnson, Naz and Rosie, Mike and Ezmine Fazal, Richie Suarez, Rick Diaz, Mike Schipps and Gary Rasmussen. And last, but certainly not least, Katherine Casey for her help with the review.

If I have forgotten anyone, please forgive me for my oversight and know I am thankful to all who helped me along the way.

FOREWORD

I have had the pleasure of knowing Ron Daniels for many years. He is passionate about helping people who find themselves in challenging and sometimes dangerous situations. When Ron asked me to write the foreword for his book, I was honored. Understanding that public safety is a community responsibility, I realized it was a chance for me to assist him in his work to make the citizens in our communities safe.

Time is the most important element when a call for help comes into a police station. How quickly the law enforcement officers respond is often the difference between life and death. Today, as police departments all over the country are forced to cut staff because of the economy, time becomes an even more critical issue. One of the benefits of Ron's book is that the information he provides can buy you extra minutes before the authorities arrive to help.

The greatest successes in making a community safe have always come when people work hand in hand with their local police. When people take seriously their need to protect themselves, their homes and loved ones, safety increases. When like-minded, safety oriented individuals come together with others in their community, neighborhoods become safer. Collectively, the community and police agencies become a team. This is a very important model for protection of the home and the community.

The key to making this community-police model work is education and observation. The police professionals study trends in criminal activity. They work closely with other important departments that provide services to citizens. Fire departments look at trends in construction of homes and how those trends increase or decrease safety in case of a fire. Public works departments trim trees and remove trash and debris so emergency vehicles have access and branches do not make contact with electrical wires.

The information these departments gather is critical knowledge for all members of the community and disseminating it in a clear, easy to understand way is crucial. Community leaders need to become involved in receiving and purveying this information in order to increase the safety of everyone.

This brings us back to the element of time. The knowledge of safety procedures, whether you are out and about or at home, will give you time to evade a dangerous situation or prevent it altogether. When Ron created The Ultimate Lock System, it meant that people could prevent home invasions. When they call for help, police have time to get to a scene and stop a crime from happening. In writing this book, Ron shares his full passion for keeping people safe in all situations. His advice will allow them to take care of themselves as individuals and to become the kind of partner to law enforcement agencies that will improve the safety of their community.

That is why a safety professional like Ron Daniels is so important. The knowledge he shares is easy to follow and will give everyone who applies it an edge when it comes to their personal safety. I would encourage everyone to read this book. Armed with its critical, life saving information, you can remain safe in this unsafe world.

—C.O. "Brad" Bradford
former Houston Chief of Police
member of Houston City Council
attorney and public safety consultant

*Courage is what preserves our liberty,
safety, life, and our homes and parents, our
country and children.*

—Plautus

It is better to be safe than sorry.

—American proverb

INTRODUCTION

Crime in the United States accounts for more deaths, injuries and loss of property than all natural disasters combined.

According to a report released by *Scientific American* magazine, one of the two major American crime epidemics occurred during the end of the 1980s and the early 1990s, during a recession. In fact, the same report related the recession and crime increase of the late 80s epidemic to the recession Americans are currently facing. In 2008, New York City saw a 54% increase in robberies. Many safety experts believe this trend will continue to carry over into smaller cities, with criminals striking homes and offices to fill the economic voids they're experiencing.

Do you feel that your personal safety is compromised? Have you ever found yourself walking through a dark alley or parking lot, fearing someone may be lurking nearby, ready to attack you? Are you worried about home invasions, crimes in which people enter your house and terrorize the owners? Are you concerned about your children or aging parents being safe?

If you answered yes to any of the above questions, this book is for you. It provides sound, professional advice on how to remain safe in an unsafe world!

I have been a police officer in Houston, Texas, for more than 10 years now. During that time, I have seen the results of hundreds of crimes directly and have heard dispatch talk on the police radio about many more. I have witnessed the devastating impact on the victims and the difficulties they have faced getting their lives back in order.

I started my life after college as an entrepreneur, but in my 30s, I decided I wanted to help people more directly and joined the Harris County Police Department. By then, I was motivated and worked hard, attaining the rank of captain more quickly than anyone else on the force before me. Along the way, I did rotations in many of the front line jobs of police officers. Patrolling some of the most dangerous areas in the city by squad car exposed me to the darkest forms of crime, including drug abuse, gang-related felonies, murders, assaults, robberies and home invasions. I discovered that there is a war going on and in many cases, our forces are woefully inadequate to hold the line against the criminals.

My heart would go out to the victims of criminal acts, who were usually ill prepared to deal with the terror that descended on them like a tornado that came out of the blue, turned their life upside down and left it in shambles. But while many had a hard time coping with what had happened, I was also impressed by their fortitude and determination to go on.

As a result, I found that I most enjoyed my rotations in education. I worked with juvenile offenders and taught crime prevention to local groups of citizens interested in taking charge of their lives. After dealing with hardened criminals, this was a welcome ray of sunshine. I felt that I had found my calling. I became passionate about helping people help themselves.

Juveniles who have been in trouble are often confused and ultimately eager to rejoin society in a positive way. Many citizens or civilians, as we members of the police force call the people who pay our salaries with their taxes, and who we ultimately work to serve and protect, are eager to help themselves and their local police in making their world a safer place.

Unfortunately, during the current recession, this is becoming problematic. As state and local governments look for ways to meet budget shortfalls, cuts in police departments make it increasingly difficult to do all the things required to combat crime. Educational programs are the first to go, followed by cops on the beat who operate on the front lines. At the same time, economic hardship leads to an increase in property crimes. It's a vicious circle with no end in sight until our economy rights itself.

With government spending cuts and a reduction in police presence in our communities, people are forced to rely more on themselves to ensure their own safety and that of their families. And while many citizens are willing to step up to the plate to do so, it is not an easy task—for most, it means starting from scratch and having to educate themselves without adequate resources.

When I thought about how to help people ensure safety in their homes, I decided to design a protective device, a high-security lock that guards against home invasions and allows families to create safe rooms inside their houses. I called it The Ultimate Lock, and you can read more about it in the Appendix to this book.

But I also realized that people need to be educated about the issues, and that they could use a resource guide of suggestions on how to cope with a variety of personal safety issues. That is why I decided to write this book, and I offer it here in the spirit of American can-do and know-how, hoping that it will allow individuals to take charge of their lives and protect themselves and their families. I believe that if we become more aware of our surroundings, follow basic rules of smart behavior and institute safety measures, we can continue to live our lives fully without constant fear and worry, secure in the knowledge that we have done everything possible to keep ourselves and our families protected.

Ron Daniels
Captain, Harris County Constables
Houston, Texas
March 2011

Chapter 1

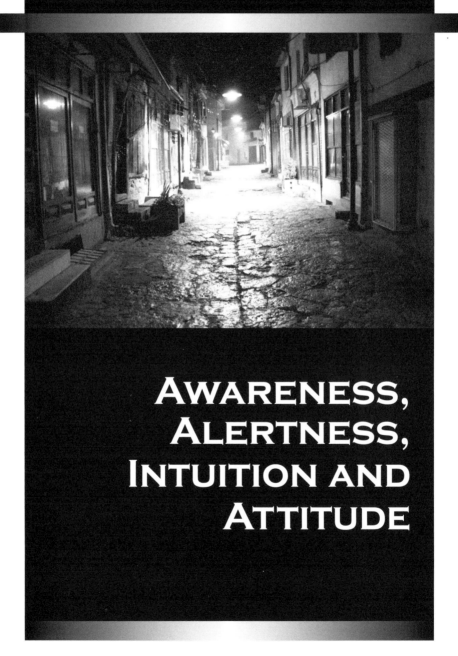

AWARENESS, ALERTNESS, INTUITION AND ATTITUDE

A reporter went out in New York City with a mugger who had recently been released from prison and was working to turn his life around. The reporter wanted to find out how criminals choose their victims. Were there any common traits of behavior that they look for in their prey?

At some point, they visited a quiet residential neighborhood. It was early afternoon and most people were at work. The tree-lined street was empty, except for a single woman who was walking in their direction on the sidewalk across from them.

The reporter nudged the ex-con, "What about her? There's no one around. Wouldn't she make a good candidate?"

But the ex-mugger shook his head and said, "No. She is aware of us."

That recognition alone—that the woman was paying attention to her surroundings—was enough for him to dismiss her as a prospective victim and look elsewhere. He preferred his prey to be easy marks—distracted, daydreaming, unfocused and unwary.

Statistics bear out that story: Those who are *aware* of their surroundings at all times are more likely to maintain their personal safety than those who go through life with their head in the clouds.

AWARENESS IS EVERYTHING

Awareness is similar to insurance. We all purchase insurance for our cars, valuables, homes and other things that matter to us. After all, we want to keep our assets secure and safe. Yet, many people fail to realize the importance of doing the same for their personal safety. Awareness—insurance for our personal well-being—is just as critical. All it takes is letting our guard down at the wrong moment to put our lives in danger.

While it's not vital to be "on guard" and expecting the worst at all times, awareness to our surroundings is crucial. Indeed, awareness will be a constant theme throughout this book. It is the cornerstone of safety, the foundation for all the other ways and recommendations we will discuss in this book for guaranteeing our personal protection. Without awareness, none of them will work successfully.

So, this is where we will begin!

Let's look at another situation, a story I heard on the police radio and remember vividly.

Candace was returning to her car in the parking lot of a large mall. She had parked farther away from the entrance that day than usual, but she was not worried. What could go wrong in broad daylight? Physically fit, she felt safe in the belief that she could call for help and take care of herself if anything happened. So when she came out of the store, she was carrying the purchases she had made in a large shopping bag and chatting with a friend on her cell phone—she failed to notice two men who were stalking her.

As they moved in her direction, another shopper spotted them and observed that they were wearing long trench coats. That struck her as odd. It was a hot, sunny day, and these men did not look like regular shoppers. She quickly called 911 on her cell phone.

Although the police responded right away, by the time they got there it was almost too late. The men had overpowered Candace, forced her into the car, and demanded she hand over her purse. When she didn't comply immediately, one of them brutally stabbed her in the side and shoved her further into the car.

The police came on the scene just as the second stalker began to attack Candace. Hearing the sirens, the criminals ran off, pursued by one of the squad cars. An ambulance arrived and took Candace to a nearby hospital where she received five stitches. She was lucky she got off so easy. The other shopper's awareness and quick thinking probably saved her life.

Lessons from Candace's ordeal

When shopping at the mall or a grocery store, try to park as close to the entrance of the building as possible. Find a busy area to park and shop—our grandmas were right when they said, "There's safety in numbers." Check out where the area's security measures are located. Many stores now have security cameras and guards patrolling the area.

As you leave the store and make your way to your car, scan the lot for other people. Take note of anyone looking suspicious or out of place. Walk with confidence and radiate awareness. Do not, I repeat, *do not* talk on your cell phone. It will distract your attention from your surroundings. If you need to make a call, wait until you have gotten into your car and *locked the doors*! If you happen to receive a call while you're still walking, ignore it until you are in a secure space.

Do not trust anyone who comes up to you and asks you a question. He may try to lure you into a trap by asking for help, trying to sell you something or requesting you to take a look at something in his car. Don't acknowledge him and get away fast. If necessary, make a big ruckus to attract attention and to deter him from pursuing you further.

When approaching your car in a lighted parking lot at night, be sure to glance underneath the vehicle. As you press the lock release button, the inside lights will turn on. Before opening the door and getting in, quickly glance inside and make sure you don't have unwelcome guests waiting for you.

The bottom line is this: Take a visual scan of the area around you whenever arriving at a new location. Observe whether anything unusual is going on. You never know! Someone might be sitting in a car down the street, waiting for his next victim. If you spot something that feels wrong and potentially dangerous, call the police. After all, you pay local taxes that fund public safety, and you should feel comfortable utilizing the services of the police department whenever necessary. Believe me, we get called to so many harrowing crime scenes, we don't mind a false alarm. And you end up being safe rather than sorry.

You should make this a regular practice for out-of-the way places, *as well as* familiar territory. It shouldn't be just a dimly lit alley or nighttime parking lot that piques your awareness and causes you to take precautions. You could be in your front yard in the middle of the day. Perhaps you are out gardening, wearing a big, wide-brim hat, taking advantage of the balmy weather, and thinking of nothing other than the flowerbed in front of you. In short, you are relaxed…too relaxed. Statistics indicate that 70% of crimes happen on the street where the victim lives! It is critical that you always use your awareness skills, no matter where you are or what you are doing.

I will be talking throughout this book about the specific things you need to be aware of in a variety of vulnerable areas and situations. While we cannot control everything around us, we can make it more difficult and challenging for criminals to choose us as their next victim.

Convey a "kick-ass" attitude

Closely related to awareness is the way you carry yourself. Always be alert—I can't say it enough! When you're alert and aware, you will find it much easier to react when something does happen. If you look like someone who knows what you're about, show awareness of your surroundings, seem to be clear about where you're headed, and walk with confidence and a "don't mess with me" attitude, more likely than not, most criminals will cut you a wide berth. They want things to be easy, to go about their business without any trouble. If you convey a "kick-ass" attitude, they'll look for someone more distracted, frailer and less aware.

LISTEN TO YOUR INNER VOICE

Have you ever felt as if you were being watched? Have you ever had the sense that something is not quite right, even if you couldn't put your finger on it? Have you ever arrived at some familiar place, only to get the feeling that something odd is going on? Perhaps you come home and a car is parked in front of your house. You notice that the driver is watching you closely. You're likely to get an eerie feeling in your gut because your body (animalistic instinct) is trying to warn you of potential danger. That is your intuition talking and putting you on high alert.

Listen to that inner voice, and pay attention to any sudden physical signs your body gives off—such as perspiring heavily, feeling flushed, experiencing constriction in your chest or stomach, or having your ears ring. These are important warning signs that may indicate possible danger. While most people ignore their natural instincts, those who trust them can often avoid precarious situations.

If your gut tells you something is wrong, do not take a chance of becoming a victim by automatically assuming that it's just your imagination and everything's fine. Trust your instincts! It is always better to err on the side of caution and safety. If you feel uneasy or anything looks out of place, call the authorities and let them investigate.

PLAN AHEAD

Cultivating an attitude of awareness also requires thinking about the future. When you find yourself in either a familiar or a new area or situation, always be aware of how you can get away in case something dangerous happens. Never put yourself in a position where you are trapped without an escape route. Look for exits. If you are in a parking lot, know which direction to run to safety.

There is great benefit in planning ahead and thinking about how you might react in specific situations. Police officers do that all the time—they run scenarios with each other and in their heads to make sure they're well prepared for any challenge or danger. Take a tip from the pros and start doing this for yourself.

Part of staying safe is always having a backup plan!

RECOGNIZE YOUR FEARS

If some of this discussion makes you feel anxious, that's okay. Knowing what situations make you uncomfortable is the first step toward learning to cope with them. The way to conquer your fears is to recognize and confront them. (We will discuss all the things you can do in greater detail in Chapter 7 on preventive measures.) For now, you can begin by looking at what other people do to feel safer in those situations. Another productive thing you can do right away is to research criminal mentality. Once you understand and become aware of how different crimes are committed, you will gain confidence that you can then use that knowledge to prevent them from happening to you.

CONCLUSION

How can you become more aware? Well, as Yogi Berra said about the great American pastime, "Baseball is 90% mental and the other half is physical." He got the mental part absolutely right. You have a choice in where to put your focus and attention. The next time you drive to the supermarket, apply what I've been talking about. Make it a habit—wherever you go—to first check out your surroundings. Whether you are at the doctor's office, a birthday party for someone else's child, a restaurant, or the local branch of your bank, start out in observation mode! Where are the entrances and exit? Is there a fire exit? How many people are there? Is there anyone who doesn't seem to belong? Are the others tense or relaxed, "into" their activities or distracted? Are they tuning out the world by listening to their iPod or aware of their surroundings?

Then ask yourself: If there were a problem, what would I do? Where would I go? How would I protect myself?

Practice this regularly, and in time, it will become second nature. Like the woman in the story at the beginning of this chapter, criminals will notice that you're aware and alert, and will think twice before choosing you as their next victim.

5 POINT PLAN

1. Be aware of your surroundings.

2. Convey a "kick-ass" attitude to the world.

3. Listen to your intuition—your inner voice—especially if something doesn't feel right

4. Plan ahead and consider how you might react in a variety of critical situations.

5. Train your mind and practice becoming more aware at all times.

Chapter 2

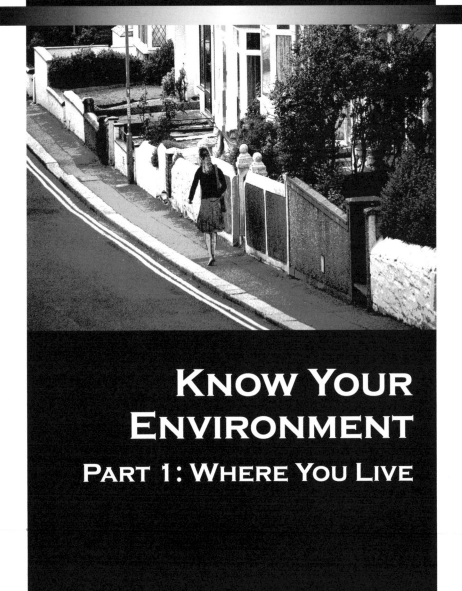

KNOW YOUR ENVIRONMENT
PART 1: WHERE YOU LIVE

Being aware is the first and most essential step for ensuring your safety. However, it is not always enough. Just as important is knowing what to pay attention to in your surroundings. Depending on where you live, work, go about your everyday activities, and attend special events, there may be a variety of issues to focus on, but when you don't know the "lay of the land," it may be more difficult to determine what are normal, as opposed to extraordinary, circumstances. You may not be aware that a gang has moved into your quiet suburban neighborhood. You may not know that robbers have targeted single women in large mall parking lots in your town. You may have just moved to a new part of the city and be unaware of the number of sex offenders who live in the area.

Perhaps the most difficult time is when you move to another town or community. You're most vulnerable in new, unfamiliar territory where you don't know the basic rules.

A few years back, in a northeastern city, a football player from a small town in Florida was mugged on his first day at college. Brian was a tall, muscular guy, confident in his physical strength and ability to take care of himself. He was wearing gold chains around his neck and was walking on a busy street two blocks away from the university campus, unaware that he was straying into the border zone of a nearby ghetto. Like an unwitting tourist, Brian was taking in the sights and not paying attention to what was happening on the street. Before he knew it, he was surrounded by five young men who put a knife to his throat and ripped the gold chains from his neck. It all happened in a matter of seconds. Fortunately, Brian wasn't hurt and sustained nothing more serious than the loss of his jewelry and the bruising of his ego. Coming from a small town where everyone knew everyone else, it hadn't occurred to him that he was now in a very different, more dangerous environment. He did use his experience as a wake-up call, however, and quickly learned to adapt to his new urban surroundings.

We are most at risk in new locales when we don't know what we don't know, and can't always identify warning signs. This is why educating yourself about the places where you live and work is critical.

In this chapter, we will look at various living environments—residential, rural, suburban and city. We will deal with workplaces and special circumstances in subsequent chapters.

RESIDENTIAL AREAS

It used to be that you could divide the country into three distinct areas—"downtown" inner city cores, surrounding suburbs and vast stretches of rural areas dotted with small towns. But over the last 30 years, central cities and suburbs have expanded and melded into metropolitan sprawls, composed of bedroom communities, small towns, strip malls and large malls, and a variety of commercial centers that often blend with residential areas. Houston, Texas, for example, has three downtown areas with high-rise buildings and skyscrapers, and a surrounding urban sprawl that includes industrial right next to residential zones which include trailer parks, condos and traditional one-house-per-property suburban tracts.

Similarly, population patterns have changed. The norm used to be largely white suburban communities with Hispanic and African-American central city cores, but this is no longer the case. Many of the traditional suburbs have as varied a population as New York City. If you live in the tri-state area of New Jersey, New York and Connecticut, or the western suburbs of Chicago, for example, you're likely to encounter a mix of white, African-American, Hispanic, and Asian-American residents, not to mention immigrants from Russia and other eastern European countries, as well as Arabs and Far East Indians. At the same time, many whites have moved back into core cities, as neighborhoods have become "gentrified."

As a result, many of the problems and crimes we used to associate only with inner cities—gangs, drugs, sex offenders, larceny, robbery and murder—have gone suburban and even spilled into rural areas.

To understand the current similarities and differences among these settings better, I have divided the discussion into three different areas:

■ **Rural:** in the country where homes and cattle, dairy or agricultural farms are often located miles away from each other. Only 20% of Americans live in these areas.

■ **High-density metropolitan:** high-rises, large apartment complexes and neighborhoods of row houses and large, three- or four-story family dwellings. (Often these houses are divided into apartments, too.)

■ **Lower-density suburban:** mostly single-family homes surrounded by yards, with some two- and three-story apartment building communities and strip malls, large malls and shopping areas of various sizes. We're going to spend most of our time with this category, as more than 50% of the U.S. population live in these low-density environments.

RURAL ENVIRONMENTS

People in what may seem like desolate areas to most of us are used to living by themselves and tend to know quickly when things are out of joint. Many isolated farms have watchdogs that draw attention to strangers immediately. Many farms now also have security systems and warning devices in place that give people who live there advance notice of arrivals when they enter the gate from the highway.

Still, it pays to be vigilant.

While on patrol, we received a call from dispatch to help a woman who had been robbed and sexually assaulted in her home. Beth lived on a rural farm estate with a heavy gate and a high fence surrounding the property. She was badly shaken up and had no idea who could have done this—her attackers had worn ski masks. At first, we could not figure out how her assailants had gotten past the gate, but when we questioned her further, it became clear what had happened. Earlier that week, she had had some repairs done to her house. Sure enough, we discovered that her spare gate opener was missing, and that led us to the culprits.

In their statements to the police, the workers later explained that the lady of the house, an attractive middle-aged woman, met them when they arrived and told them that she didn't have time to talk to them. Her husband usually handled matters that concerned the upkeep of the house, but he was out of town on a business trip. She left the repairmen to go about their business upstairs unattended and spent the time with a female friend in the sitting room downstairs. The workers noticed jewelry on the night stand in the bedroom, as well as skimpy lingerie on the floor. A quick search of the drawers of her makeup table yielded the spare gate opener. When they were finished, Beth just waved good-bye from the den and continued her conversation with her friend. The next day, the workers and members of the gang they belonged to decided to pay her a visit.

If you live in a rural town and you have repairs done to your home or have furniture or appliances delivered, make sure you supervise or pay close attention. Don't leave strangers alone in any part of the house. You never know what they might notice that sparks their interest. Even if they themselves aren't potential criminals, they might tell someone else what they observed, and that person could decide to make you his target.

High-density metropolitan environments

Although outsiders consider big cities especially dangerous, they are often safer than medium-sized towns and smaller communities because the former have the benefit of an active street life. There are many retail stores, bars and other venues open 24 hours a day, where people can go in case of trouble.

City dwellers know to avoid certain neighborhoods, especially after dark, and to steer clear of unlit areas and alleys. If they take the subway late at night, they tend to congregate in one or two cars, usually close to the front of the train where the conductor is, while the rest of the train remains empty. They know that there is relative safety in numbers.

They also know how to wear "city armor," by projecting a combination of awareness and a "don't mess with me" attitude. They won't look directly in the eyes of people they pass on the street, because that is an invitation to get approached and hassled. Instead, they glance at them out of the corner of their eyes, and move on with determination.

They know that underground parking garages for high-rise apartment buildings and condos are vulnerable areas. Many will have concierges or guards at the entrance, making it less likely that unauthorized people will gain access.

Still, there are a large number of unattended buildings. If you live in one of them, make sure that you don't get into an elevator alone with someone you don't know. When you open the downstairs door or gate, don't let someone you don't know come in with you, like a well-dressed stranger who claims to have lost his keys or is "just" visiting someone. Let him ring the doorbell or call the building superintendent on his own.

If he forces his way inside, get as quickly as you can to the guard or night watchman on duty. Make a scene if you can. Better safe than sorry. In such situations, it helps to have your phone on speed dial to the police or building management so you can call them right away.

It is useful to get to know your super and guards by name, so that when you see someone you don't know behind the desk, you can find out why. Many guards are provided by security services and rotate or fill in when someone is out sick. If, for some reason, there is a new guard on duty who makes you feel uncomfortable or tries to follow you into your residence, call 911 and have him checked out. He could be a decoy. If he is a legitimate backup guard, it is better to apologize than to pay the price for not listening to your intuition and following through on a hunch.

LOW-DENSITY SUBURBAN ENVIRONMENTS

Although these suburbs are where most Americans live today, they are anything but uniform. In some suburban communities, the houses are so close to one another that you can virtually see into your neighbor's kitchen or bedroom. In others, you may be on a two-acre property, well set back from the road with your "next-door" neighbor's house barely visible behind some trees. You may live in a gated community with security guards that need to be contacted before visitors are granted entrance. (Often the guards will take down names of the occupants and license plate numbers of the cars that arrive.) Or, you may have an apartment or condo in a "village" composed of a number of two- or three-story buildings. Some of these housing developments have a security guard at the front entrance. Many do not.

Something all of these suburban communities share, however, is open space—whether it's a park, athletic facility or backyard with bushes and trees—where criminals can hide.

Ashley, a young mom, was attending her son Timmy's afternoon baseball practice in a large athletic park that had a playground and soccer, football and baseball fields with bleachers and dugouts. When practice was over, people started to head home, but Timmy wanted to practice and play some more. Against her better judgment, Ashley stayed behind with him by herself.

Soon it got dark. When Timmy couldn't find his ball and went to look for it under the bleachers, he encountered three men. One of them had his ball and another carried a baseball bat. Ashley instantly recognized that they meant trouble. She felt helpless not knowing what to do and wished she had gone home with the other parents.

Just then, the father of one of her son's teammates drove up. The boy, realizing he had taken Timmy's glove by mistake, had asked his dad to turn around and drive back. When the headlights illuminated the bleachers, the three men walked away.

Ashley and Timmy were very lucky.

Avoid parks and deserted areas if you are alone, even during the day, but especially in the evening hours and late at night. We will discuss later what to do if you get in trouble (Chapters 8 and 9), but it's best not to be caught there by yourself in the first place.

PAY ATTENTION IN SHOPPING PARKING LOTS

Anytime you go to a bank, grocery store, mall or a dimly lit area, always stop to think for a moment. Do you feel safe? Business owners are becoming more aware that their customers require security and safety measures in order for them to shop without concern. You should look for shopping centers where adjustments have been made accordingly—parking lots with lights, and cameras and security guards monitoring the area. If you have any concerns, do not get out of your car. When you do leave your automobile, quickly move to a safe area inside the mall. Listen to your "inner voice" and pay attention to any physical signs your body gives off, indicating possible danger.

BE ALERT COMING HOME

Pay attention when coming home alone, especially at night. I stress this because many people automatically feel safe on their own property or in familiar surroundings and let their guard down. Yet, each year millions of crimes take place right in the victim's own driveway! Being in law enforcement, I have been called to many crime scenes where people thought they were safe in their garage or the lot of their apartment building, but as soon as they stepped out of their car, they were mugged, assaulted or hurt.

Janet, a young, attractive woman, was carrying her groceries up the outside stairs to the second floor of the condo building where she lived. It was late at night, and although there was ample lighting, it did not deter two members of a gang from approaching her menacingly.

What they hadn't counted on was that Janet kept a small air horn in her purse. As they closed in on her with switchblades drawn, ready to shove her to the ground, she managed to pull it out and squeezed the trigger. The sound blast not only stopped them in their tracks, it brought out every tenant in the building looking for what had made that noise. When doors flew open upstairs and downstairs, the criminals took off as fast as they could.

Janet was understandably shaken, but she had stood her ground. I can't tell you how proud we were of her after being called to the scene and finding out what had happened.

In another case, a woman pulled into her garage late at night. Melissa's house was empty—her teenage children were away—and she was about to get out of the car with her shopping bags when she noticed in the rearview mirror that the garage door hadn't closed although she had pushed the remote.

Melissa immediately locked the doors. She had OnStar in the car and pressed the emergency button. It was a good thing, because by then two young men had entered the garage and were smashing her car windows, trying to get at her. Somehow, she managed to put the car in reverse and back out fast, hitting one of the men with her rear bumper. The other man chased after her, but Melissa slammed the car into forward and drove off. OnStar was with her on the line the whole way and notified the police.

When we got to the house, we noticed a small trail of blood on the driveway from the man she had hit. We located him quickly, because he had only managed to limp a few blocks—his partner had disappeared, however. The assailant claimed that he had just been out walking in the neighborhood and that the woman had run him down as he was passing by. When we took him to the station and investigated further, we discovered that he lived more than 12 miles away and was a convicted felon who had been in prison for just this type of crime—robbing unsuspecting drivers in their garage.

Once again, it was awareness and quick thinking and reacting that saved Melissa from harm.

To protect yourself, even in your own "safe" driveway, try not to leave yourself exposed for extended amounts of time. When you are bent over in your car, unpacking groceries in the backseat while the garage door is open, you won't be able to see who may be lingering behind you. If there is someone at home already, it's best to call ahead and let him or her know that you are coming. Perhaps they can turn on the porch light and watch for your arrival. Wait for the garage door to open, drive inside and immediately close the door before exiting your car. Make sure you stay in the car until the garage door is completely closed and you can be sure no one has followed you.

If something unusual occurs, keep your car locked and begin to back out of the garage immediately. For instance, you might notice that the garage door as it's closing stops partway and goes back up. This can be a warning sign that someone is trying to get into the garage with you, as many garage doors have motion detectors nowadays and will start to open again if they sense movement (a safety measure to prevent accidents from happening, such as children playing and getting their arms or legs trapped beneath the closing door). That is why it is extremely important to stay in the car until you are certain you're safe.

You should apply the same caution when leaving the garage. Get in the car, lock the doors, have your cell phone available, start the car, and put the transmission in reverse before you open the garage door. Criminals who have cased your house and know your schedule may be waiting outside the garage and try to run in as soon as the door starts to open. If you're not ready to leave, they might have enough time to attack you. If you are in the car with the doors locked, the car running and ready to back out of the garage, you can move quickly. If you see someone suspicious lingering, back out quickly without stopping, get on the street and call the authorities on your cell phone as you are driving away.

ADDITIONAL TIPS TO HELP YOU STAY SAFE

Do not put your name on your mailbox. These days, criminals are getting creative. They may appear in UPS or FedEx uniforms, impersonating deliverymen, pretending to deliver a package. Or they may come to your front door and say, "I have a letter here for Mrs. So-and-so." You'll be lulled into a false sense of security and end up mugged, robbed or worse.

If you are outside gardening or sunning yourself by the swimming pool, pay attention. Unless you live in a gated community, you never know who might be coming by—from the electrical company representative reading the meter to strangers passing through the neighborhood.

If you live in a dark area where houses are far apart, invest in a security system and lights that can illuminate the environment.

You may also want to install a sensor near the gate or front of your driveway so you have ample warning about anyone approaching your house by car or truck. There have been cases of robbers driving up with a U-Haul to the front door of a house off the road and cleaning the place out. The neighbors, a few hundred yards away, thought the owners were moving and didn't alert the police.

If you live on a poorly lit street and notice strange people coming and going in the neighborhood, or if you hear that someone was attacked and the criminals used the darkness to their advantage, be proactive. Go to the hardware store and get an automatic security light, which activates by motion when anybody gets near the house. Perhaps criminals will then pass up your house because they are not comfortable taking a chance where they can be seen or caught.

Criminals try to make you think everything is OK in order to set you up for a fall. They will case you, your car, your jewelry, and your habits—when you come and go and where you are going. They may be out in the open where they can be seen every day, for weeks at a time. You get used to them being around and become relaxed.

In one instance, a group of criminals monitored the routine of a woman for more than a month without her becoming suspicious. As a manager in the corporate office for a chain of convenience stores, Rachel drove a nice car, was always well dressed and wore expensive jewelry. The gang learned that she left for work at a certain time in the morning and left her place of work in the afternoon at the same time each day to make deposits at the same bank. The criminals knew that she was handling the deposits and operating cash for 22 stores. They also discovered that her routine included a midday stop to pick up her daughter from preschool and take her home to a babysitter.

When the criminals were ready, they staged an accident on her way to the bank, and when Rachel got out of the car, surrounded her and threatened her with guns. They demanded the bag that contained the money to be deposited and told her that they knew what time she picked up her daughter and would hurt them both if she talked to the police. As a result, Rachel refused to cooperate with us because she feared retaliation, and the robbers were never caught. Since she had not been aware of them before, she was now paranoid and thought they were secretly watching her at all times.

CONCLUSION

You do not need to become paranoid, but you do need to be aware of what is happening around you. You need to understand when to walk or drive in another direction, and to vary your pattern of behavior so that it can't be used against you.

5 POINT PLAN

1. Do not leave repairmen or other strangers unattended in your home.

2. Avoid dark, unlit areas at night—be they alleys, parking lots, athletic facilities or other unattended areas.

3. Make sure your garage door is closed before you exit your vehicle to go into the house.

4. Similarly, be ready to drive off as soon as your garage door opens.

5. Change your routine, whether it is going to work and coming home or making deliveries during the day.

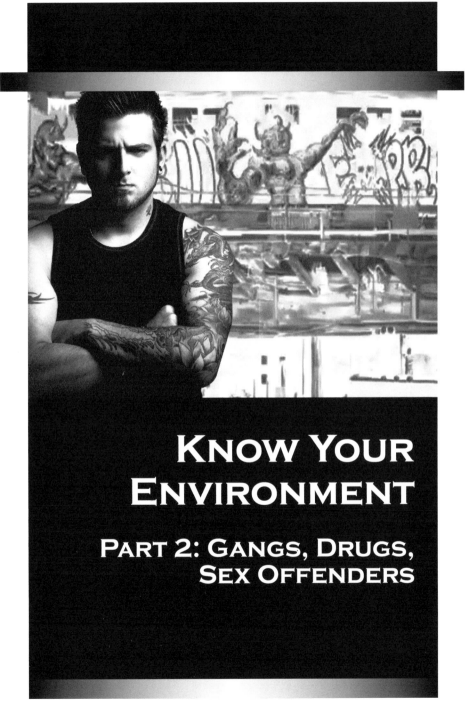

Know Your Environment

Part 2: Gangs, Drugs, Sex Offenders

As I mentioned earlier, many of the problems we used to associate with inner cities—gangs, drugs, sex offenders—have traveled to suburbia and even spilled into rural areas.

How do you know that your community is beset with such problems? Well, nowadays, it is almost a given that drug usage and drug dealing take place in one or more areas or neighborhoods in the town where you live. The question for you is how to best find out where, so you can avoid such places or know how to deal with them.

STAY INFORMED REGARDING THE NEWS

Do you watch the morning or evening news on television? Do you read the daily newspaper in your city? If you do, you already know that the level of violence on the streets is increasing. While many citizens don't inform themselves, preferring to remain blissfully ignorant, I don't recommend that you become one of them. Staying updated regarding what's going on around you by watching the local news and reading the newspaper is an excellent way to begin to protect yourself. You will have a good idea of what the level of violence in your area is, what you should be on the lookout for, and how you can better guard against being a victim of common crimes.

VISIT YOUR LOCAL POLICE DEPARTMENT

If you're new to the area, go to your local police department and ask to speak to someone who can tell you all about your community and what you may want to watch out for. Many police departments have liaison officers for just this purpose. Ask about recent crimes that have occurred. If you are looking to move into an apartment complex, find out the crime statistics for that property. Look at the reports and check what the police response time was. If you have children, find out about the schools that are in the better parts of town. Even if you can't afford to live in the more upscale neighborhoods, many communities make it possible for students to attend a variety of schools in the system. Take a look at all the schools your child may attend and determine if there is gang activity in any of them. Base your final decision for enrollment on all the information you have gathered.

To protect yourself fully, you'll need to understand the methods by which local criminals ply their trade—what seems to be their *modus operandi* or mode of operation (MO), as we call it in law enforcement. You may be asking yourself, "How could I possibly understand their way of doing things?" Remember, I'm not asking you to study criminal behavior in exquisite detail. But, if you saw in the local paper that women in your area are being attacked in parking lots of grocery stores (pushing carts to the car or having both hands occupied with grocery bags makes people more vulnerable), you would be more aware when returning to your vehicle after shopping. If you know that home invasions are on the rise in your community, you can take measures to protect yourself and your family.

It's likely that what you see on the news and read about will only reveal some of the areas criminals are targeting. But that will give you an understanding of the types of avenues they are pursuing to gain unlawful advantage.

So it is critical for you to stay updated and ahead of the curve. You want to be prepared for any and all possibilities. Make your family and children aware of what is happening in your area as well. There could be information about someone riding around in a van targeting small children. You need to explain to your children what to do if they encounter this type of situation, so they might be able to save their lives or their friends' lives.

Being well informed will also help you with the three banes of contemporary American life, much in the news: gangs, sex offenders and drugs.

UNDERSTAND GANG BEHAVIOR

There are gangs in every city of the United States. If you think for a moment, you can likely name a few streets or neighborhoods in your town where gang activity occurs. Being aware of these areas, staying out of them, or moving through them quickly may save your life. In addition, if you know the MO of gangs, you can avoid certain dangerous situations.

Let's talk a bit about what the attraction of gangs is for those who join them, what characterizes their behavior, and why they would go out of their way to hurt innocent people.

Many gang members have poor self-esteem. They feel that they've never had anyone who cares for them. They have witnessed so many murders occurring in their neighborhoods that violence and killing seem to be a routine part of life. Gang leaders attract members by providing protection from this everyday reality. They will offer money to recruits or buy them new clothes to try to show them they care. The prospective member sees this as a "way out" and accepts the family atmosphere of the gang without realizing that it is all trickery, and that the leaders only want to grow their gang's size.

After joining, the new recruits are required to commit criminal acts as an initiation before becoming fully recognized members. It's important for them to "prove" themselves to their peers, and they may do so by carrying out a random drive-by shooting, firing indiscriminately into a crowd, or committing a more targeted crime involving a specific victim to rob, rape and/or kill. Because they did not have fine things growing up, new gang members are easily convinced that they should take revenge on those who do have those things.

Something else you should know is that gangs thrive on fear. They get their notoriety from all the stories in the media about the ugly things they do to other human beings. They use their high public profile of disrepute to let other gangs and the public know, "This is our territory, and if you come here, the same thing will happen to you!" What you need to understand is that these gangs want to make a name for themselves at your expense, if you give them the opportunity.

Sometimes gang members will try to bait people by flashing their car lights at you, for example. If you flash back, you immediately become their next target. They will turn around, follow you and try to stop you, with the intent of assaulting you or damaging your car.

There are several stereotypes of gang members that can be misleading. You may think from watching television that they only wear baggy pants, T-shirts, bandanas, oversized NFL jackets, and sport lots of tattoos. Sure, some do; but others are clean-shaven and well dressed, and their long-sleeved shirts may hide their tattoos. You just can't tell anymore by what someone's wearing if he is a gang member or not.

It is still true that many gangs mark their territory with graffiti on the sides of buildings and sidewalks. If you see such signs in an area unfamiliar to you, beware!

While we are discussing gangs, let's talk about "gang shoppers." These are gangs who shop for the "right victim." It's not that they're seeking out a specific age or a specific nationality (although they may be looking for a woman rather than a man, or vice versa). They are looking for anyone who fits the category they have conceived in their minds as their next victim. They are not concerned with the consequences of what they are going to do; they only care about how they can gain points for their gang membership. They want to be known for their gang association and name, not their individual identities.

If you want to avoid gang-related crime, don't put yourself into circumstances where you're seen as easy prey. Use common sense, be alert and be aware. The best thing to do is to stay out of their area of influence.

SHOULD YOU STOP OR SHOULD YOU RUN?

What if you happen to venture into gang territory accidently? Or what if you're walking down the street and are approached by strangers who make you feel uncomfortable? Or what if at night you find yourself on a dimly lit street, and something does not feel right to you?

Get your cell phone out and call 911 immediately! Let the dispatcher know you are in a potentially bad situation. Give as much information as possible about where you are, how many people are nearby and their description. Just hearing you calling for help on the phone may discourage the criminals and save your life.

Most criminals are quite concerned with rousing the authorities, so they may think twice before getting involved with you. They know where the boundary line lies between getting away with something and getting caught. Your job is to make them believe that when they mess with you they'll be stepping over that line.

BE AWARE OF SEX OFFENDERS

Another criminal element that requires your awareness is sex offenders. Convicted sex offenders sometimes live right on your street or close to the schools your children attend. There are now websites developed by local law enforcement officials in every state, where you can look up if there are any pedophiles living in your neighborhood, and find out their names, addresses, what type of sex crimes they were charged with, and what age group of children they target.

Some police departments even send out notices through the mail when a sex offender moves into an area. This is important information if your children have to wait for the bus in the morning to take them to school and come home by bus in the afternoon. In some areas it may be necessary for parents to team up and take turns to wait with the grade school-age children in the morning and pick them up at the bus stop later in the day. The same watchful attitude and measures go for playgrounds in the neighborhood.

You need to understand what methods sex offenders use to lure youngsters into a bad situation, so you can explain to your children how they can protect themselves when they are on their own. Sexual deviates may ask for help or directions in an attempt to get close enough to grab a child. They may try to lure their victims to their car with candy, puppies or other child-friendly materials. Show your children pictures of the sex offenders in your community and tell them to let you know if they see anyone who looks like that hanging around the playground or schoolyard.

If any of these deviates do show up where the children play, notify the police immediately. Make note of the make and color of their cars, license plate numbers, and description of their clothing—and anything else the police can use to identify and watch out for them in the area. If one of them comes near you, or you feel uncomfortable or threatened, call 911 immediately. In fact, if you are in a place where you know that you might encounter such criminals, keep your cell phone handy with 911 on speed dial and if one of them approaches you, tell them that you have the police on the phone, and to stay away from you.

Make sure you are aware of any unusual circumstances or incidents that have occurred in your neighborhood. Keep in mind that homes of sex offenders will often have a lot of cars and visitors at odd hours of the day and night. These may be people dealing drugs or friends who in many cases are also sex offenders.

There are now strict guidelines to make the public aware when sex offenders are present in a school district. However, sometimes these situations are not reported immediately. You want to make sure you keep yourself updated on the most recent information.

I cannot stress enough how important it is for you to be vigilant regarding this issue. When children are molested and violated, they are robbed of their childhood forever.

BE COGNIZANT OF DRUGS

Drugs have become an unfortunate part of life in just about every community in the United States. They are easily available to adults and minors. Many students—from grade school to high school—go to class high on everything from marijuana to cocaine, acid (LSD), and oxycontin (oxycodone). Various date rape drugs have been part of the singles scene for some time. The parts of town where these narcotics are sold are often high crime areas, and avoiding them is the best way to stay safe.

All too often, the problem is closer to home. Even if you've made sure that your home is safe, you should not take for granted that your child won't encounter drugs in school or when she visits friends or classmates.

In one instance, we were called to a house where a little girl on a visit had become very sick. When we and the EMS crew arrived, we discovered that she had been given sexual stimulant drugs by the uncle of her girlfriend. His intention was to rape the little girl without her being able to remember what had happened to her, but his plan backfired when he gave her too much. She had to be rushed to the hospital and have her stomach pumped. Needless to say, the uncle was caught. But how many others fall victim to such crimes and have no recourse?

The first time your child is asked to sleep over at a friend's house for a slumber party, meet the parents and stay in close contact with her—cell phones are quite useful in these situations. Make sure that there are arrangements to have her picked up immediately and returned home if she feels unsafe for any reason.

KNOW HOW TO DEAL WITH STREET VIOLENCE

Related to drug and gang activity is another type of crime that we in the police force call "street violence." This is a situation that can look perfectly normal to anyone passing by without realizing that serious trouble is brewing, yet escalate into violence in a matter of seconds. Perhaps you are sitting on your front porch, and you see a bunch of kids playing basketball and having a good time. Then, another group arrives, claiming, "Hey, this is our territory," and trying to cause trouble. All of a sudden, guns are blazing, and both the people involved and bystanders are injured or killed by stray bullets.

Once again, I cannot stress enough that we all need to be aware! Such things can happen at a moment's notice, and if you are not paying attention to what is happening around you, you or a family member could be hurt. Your child could be having a great time watching a baseball game, not realizing that the field is close to a gang neighborhood, and a stray bullet could harm him. You must inform your children of dangerous areas and insist they stay away from them. Make sure they understand to get away as soon as they see any signs of violence. They need to understand that things can get out of hand very quickly and that they do not want to be around when matters escalate.

If you happen to see incidents of violence, call the police. Many people who are eyewitnesses to crimes and violence do not want to get involved. They are afraid that they or their family might be at risk if any of the perpetrators find out they cooperated with the police. Such fears are understandable, but there are things you can do without putting yourself at risk. At least make an anonymous phone call to the authorities and let them know what is happening or has happened. Hit *67 on your cell phone or house phone to block your caller ID and make the call. No one will know who you are, and you can do your part to keep your community safe.

There are also other simple things you can do to attack crime in your area. For example, if you notice graffiti on fences or buildings in your neighborhood where they haven't been before, it may be a sign that a gang is trying to expand its territory and lay claim to the area. Instead of ignoring it, paint over the spray can "art." You'll be sending the gang members a signal that your neighborhood will not tolerate any nonsense. Follow up by posting signs offering a reward to anyone who can identify the people producing these graffiti, promising that he or she will remain anonymous. If the residents of a neighborhood band together, much good can be accomplished.

CONCLUSION

Remember, in order to be as safe as you can, it's important to know what to pay attention to in these environments and to be prepared for any and all contingencies. Knowledge is power—the power to take the necessary measures to remain safe and secure in today's world.

5 POINT PLAN

1. Inform yourself of the kind of crimes being perpetrated in your part of town by watching television and reading local newspapers.

2. Understand the way gangs operate and avoid their turf.

3. Make sure you know who the convicted sex offenders are in your neighborhood and where they live.

4. Make sure your children understand the dangers of drugs at school and in their friends' homes.

5. Counter any signs of gang encroachment like graffiti with an active neighborhood response.

Chapter 4

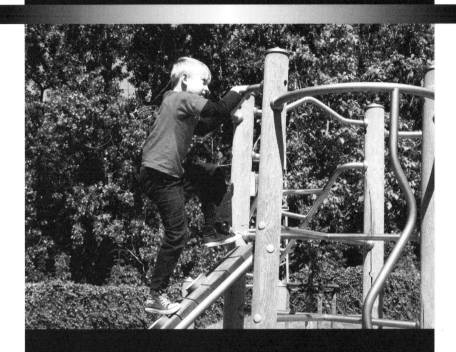

KNOW YOUR ENVIRONMENT

PART 3: WORK AND PLAY

Emily, a science teacher in an inner city high school, was working late grading lab reports. The room was on the first floor of an old brick school building. There was one door that opened into the classroom, and it had a glass viewing pane at eye level. When she heard a noise, she got up and took a look in the hallway outside the door, but no one was there. Emily closed and locked her door.

Suddenly, there was a crash and clatter of glass as a rock came hurtling through one of the windows. When Emily went over to check, there was another, bigger crash, only this time it came from the door. She turned just in time to see three teenage kids coming after her through the door they had kicked in.

Emily recognized one of the students, an 11th grader, and it was clear to her that he and his friends meant to do her harm. As she backed away behind one of the lab tables, she noticed a beaker out of the corner of her eye. It was from an experiment she had done earlier that day with her students and it still contained liquid. Without thinking she picked it up and flung it at her assailants. It was acid and it burned.

The kids started to scream, turned tail and ran away. Emily was mortified, but recovered quickly and called the police. They had no difficulty tracking down the culprits who had lost some of the skin on their faces and hands. It turned out that all three were students at the school, and members of a gang. As part of their initiation, they were ordered to assault Emily because it was known she liked to stay late and would be alone.

It was fortunate that she was quick thinking and willing to stand up for herself. One of the important lessons of this story is to use whatever you can get your hands on, whatever will give you a fighting chance, to get out of harm's way.

It is well known that over the last 20 years, teaching has become an increasingly dangerous profession. In many inner city schools, students have to pass through metal detectors in the morning to make sure they're not bringing weapons into the building. Middle and high school teachers have been assaulted, raped and killed.

But other workplaces have become more dangerous as well. Indeed, any building open to the public for retail commerce and other services is vulnerable to criminal activity, especially if money transactions frequently take place there. Even businesses like doctors' or dentists' offices and law firms are not immune when disgruntled employees return to seek revenge for being let go or fired, or when escaped convicts look to take hostages. Whether it is a suburban bank, a post office, or a city retail shop for clothes, shoes and food, you may find yourself in a hazardous situation either as an employee or as a customer.

WHAT TO DO IF YOU ARE HELD UP AT WORK

Incidents of bank robberies are on the rise again because of the recession, although the perpetrators no longer come in like Bonnie and Clyde, brandishing guns and shotguns. More than likely, the robber will walk to a teller with a note that reads something like, "I have a gun, give me your money." Tellers are instructed to hand over the money, even if the robber is not showing a weapon, as insurance companies will reimburse the loss. But make no mistake, a bank holdup is a high-tension situation, and the slightest cough or glitch can trigger—sometimes literally—a life-threatening response on the part of the robber. If he is armed and starts shooting, you don't want to get caught in the crossfire.

So, if you are an employee or customer in a store or place of business, take the time to think ahead and plan what you would do:

■ Use your awareness to "case the joint."

■ Ask yourself, where are entrances and exits, and emergency exits?

■ It there a safe room where you can go and lock the door to wait until the coast is clear?

■ Finally, keep your antennas tuned for any unusual signs and situations. There is a routine to work, and any break in it needs your attention—different sounds, people behaving oddly, people hurrying, moving too quickly.

You don't need to be on red alert all the time, but make sure you're ready.

If you happen to get caught in a holdup, stay calm and do what the robber says. That is the best way to survive such a situation without getting harmed. Whether you are an employee or customer, be sure to take note of the robber's facial features, clothing, height, weight and anything else the police can use to catch the criminal.

If you work in an office and a stranger or angry co-worker comes in with a rifle or gun, try to get to a safe room and lock the door. Wait out the assault until the police arrive. Usually, the disgruntled employee will be going after the higher-ups he thinks are responsible for his problems. But realize that he is in a chaotic emotional state and out of control, so you don't ever want to be in his sight lines.

BE AWARE IN PUBLIC ARENAS

Crowded places like the subway, a bus or the airport, or sporting events and concerts, are a paradise for pickpockets and thieves. Be prepared for people bumping into you, but don't assume it is because of the congested environment. You could be the unwitting target of a pickpocket and lose money, credit cards and other important IDs. Sometimes thieves will operate in pairs: one "accidentally" knock into you for distraction while the other lifts your wallet or purse from your pocket or handbag. Often, people don't realize they've been victimized until they attempt to make a purchase and notice their money is missing. By this time, the perpetrator is long gone.

If you're a man, carry your wallet in your front pocket rather than in back. While some rear pockets have buttons to close them up, wily thieves have been known to use knives to slash them open.

Women should hold on to their purses and handbags, or keep the wallets that hold important documents in a pouch tied around their waist like a belt. In fact, I recommend that women take fewer personal items with them in their purse when they go shopping or on an outing to a public event. When my wife goes to the grocery store, she always takes a smaller purse that contains only one credit card and her ID. That way, if—heaven forbid—she ever got mugged, she could easily cancel the card with one phone call.

Be sure never to leave purses and packages unattended in public places.

In one case, a woman dropping her young daughter off at an after-school program left her purse on the seat of her car while she went inside the building. Having locked the doors, she thought it was safe. After all, she was only going to be gone for a minute or so. But when she returned, she saw that someone had smashed the window and grabbed her purse, which contained her credit cards, social security card and other identification. She felt so shocked and embarrassed that she didn't report the crime until 24 hours later, by which time the culprit had rung up close to $90,000 in charges!

Conclusion

Keep in mind that the process of dealing with the theft of credit cards and identity documents is long and tedious. You must first call the police and give a detailed report. Next you have to call your credit card companies and put a stop on your cards and begin the process of replacing them. Then, you have to get a new driver's license, social security card, etc. Nowadays, with the heightened level of identity theft security and the questions and procedures required, this process can become a nightmare (see Chapter 13 on what to do in case you become a victim of identity theft).

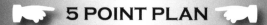

5 POINT PLAN

1. Plan ahead for how to deal with a disturbance in a public place.

2. Look for exits and safe areas to wait out the situation.

3. If you get caught in a holdup, stay calm and do what the robber says.

4. Be aware of thieves and pickpockets in crowded environments.

5. Carry your purse or wallet in a safe place.

Chapter 5

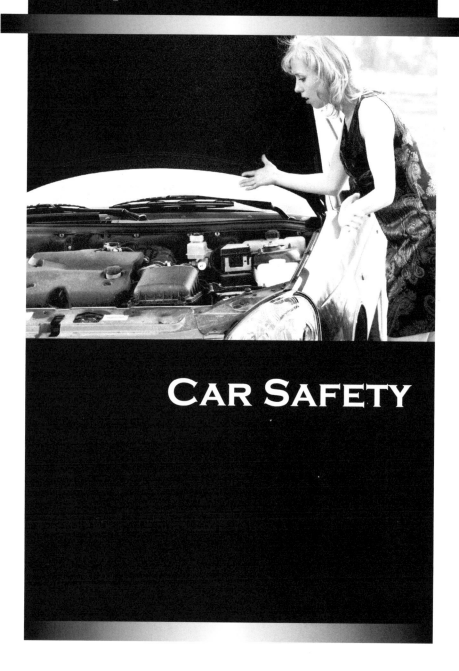

CAR SAFETY

With the development of large-scale suburbs, the automobile has become the primary form of transportation for most people in the United States. From going to work, to shopping, taking kids to school or ferrying them to various activities, visiting friends, going out for dinner, and taking vacations, the car is as much an important part of our lives as computers and cell phones. Indeed, on average, Americans spend five hours a day driving!

When people think of car safety, they usually focus on wearing seatbelts, having designated drivers for people who have had too much to drink at a dinner or party, and obeying speed limits and other traffic regulations. All that is important, of course, but just as critical is making sure you're safe in and around your vehicle before, during and after whatever trip you're taking.

Consider this scenario, for example. It is nighttime and you're on your way home from a late meeting at the office. You come upon a car on a deserted section of the road with its emergency lights flashing. The driver is outside of the car waving, attempting to flag you down. Wanting to be helpful, you decide to stop and see if you can be of assistance. What you don't know is that the driver is a decoy. At the last light, a spotter identified you as a potential victim and called ahead for him to stage the scene of a breakdown, and his fellow criminals are in hiding nearby, waiting for you to stop. As you, the unsuspecting, good Samaritan, get out of your car, they surround you, mug and rob you, or worse.

If you encounter such a situation, it would be better to call for help. Do not stop! Use your cell phone to call 911 and give the authorities the location of the driver with the broken down vehicle. Let the police handle the matter. You don't want to make yourself vulnerable, especially at night. If the stranded motorist is a decoy with partners in crime, they could be "gang shoppers" as discussed in an earlier chapter, and you do not want to be on their shopping list.

BE ALERT WHEN GETTING GAS

If you run low on gas, you may have the choice between a less expensive, dimly lit station on a side street or a brightly lit station on a main street, which charges a few cents more per gallon. Where should you go? Obviously, the brightly lit station is the better choice. While you may pay a little more at the pump, you will also minimize your risk.

Further, prepare yourself as you step out of the car by keeping your cell phone in your hand, ready to dial 911. When possible, get back into your car and lock the door while the gas is pumping—many stations have nozzles that allow you to "lock" the handle so that gas flows automatically. When the tank is full, they click off on their own. Follow the same routine with your cell phone—ready to call for help—when you get out of your car to remove the nozzle and close your gas tank. By being aware and alert, making wise choices regarding where you stop, being prepared to call for help and being proactive by locking the car door while pumping gas, you will minimize the potential dangers during your pit stop.

WHAT TO DO IF YOU'RE BEING FOLLOWED

Let's say you're pulling out of a gas station that criminals have staked out, shopping for a new victim. They watch you leave and follow you. Then they pull up beside you to check you out. Soon, another car comes up on the other side and sandwiches you between it and the other vehicle. It is important that you are aware and understand what is happening. Is it just a coincidence, or are these people trying to make you feel anxious and panic you? If it doesn't feel right, get on your cell phone right away and let someone know what is happening.

Meanwhile, make sure you stay on the main traffic artery. Do not allow yourself to get run off the road or forced to take a deserted side street. Drive to a well-lit area immediately; find a spot with many people or a lot of cars. Better yet, stop at a police or fire station. The criminals will not follow you into these "safe zones."

ERRATIC DRIVING BEHAVIOR

Suppose you're driving down an unlit road and ahead you see another car swerving back and forth. Your instincts alert you to be cautious—perhaps you're dealing with a drunken driver. It's better to hang back a little rather than accelerate immediately to try to race past him. If you do decide to move ahead and the other car accelerates to keep up with you, you know you may have a problem on your hands.

Driving erratically on purpose, criminals will often try to involve their victims in some sort of accident. They may bump you from behind or brush you from the side. When you stop and get out of your car, you become vulnerable and they will try to take advantage of you.

Again, head for a police station, fire station or a well-lit area. If you have to, use your cell phone to let the authorities know where you are and try to meet up with a patrol car. Once you've reached a safe area, report the other driver to the police, describing his vehicle's make and color, and the direction in which he was headed.

If another automobile hits you or stops suddenly in front of you so that you can't avoid rear-ending it, never get out of your car in a dark or quiet area. Always drive to a well-lit spot, where there are other people. Call 911 before getting out of the car. Be sure to inform the other driver that you've already dialed for police assistance. You never know who the other person is or why he ran into you or stopped short in front of you. However, if he knows the police are already on their way, it will minimize the chances of him attacking you.

Hit-and-run crimes

Thousands of hit-and-run accidents occur each year throughout the United States. Leaving the scene of an accident is a crime, and those who are caught will be charged accordingly. If you're the victim of such a crime, how you react in the moments after the accident is vital. Things can happen quickly and the other car may speed away before you even realize what's happening.

Obviously, the first thing to do is to assess your physical well-being and call 911. If you can, try to remember the license plate number of the other car. Short of that, note the make, model and color, and any other details—is the car a two-door or four-door model; how many passengers are inside; is the driver male or female? Does it have any damage, such as a broken window or dented door? The more information you can provide to the police, the easier it will be for them to find and apprehend the criminal. Often witnesses may stop and be able to help you fill in the gaps regarding things you didn't notice.

In the meantime, you can practice memorizing license plate numbers and telling details of other cars during your trips when you have to wait at a stoplight, for example. Develop the habit ahead of time and you'll be well prepared in case something serious does happen.

Consider an auto safety course

Do you know how to steer if one of your tires has a blowout? Or if your car starts running in an erratic manner? Or when the road is icy and you go into a skid? If not, you could potentially hurt someone or get into a bad accident because you're unfamiliar with what you can do in such emergency situations. As law enforcement officers, we take courses that train us to operate our police cars on a higher level of safety because we face unpredictable circumstances on a daily basis and have to be able to control our cars at all times, even at high speeds during a chase. You may want to enroll in a police-taught, enhanced auto safety course yourself to help you better respond to emergency situations on the road. As someone who always champions better preparedness, I believe taking such a course is a great idea. At the end of the program, you may not be able to pull off stunts, make fancy U-turns or slide into a parking spot like you see in movies and commercials, but you will feel more empowered and confident in your abilities to stay safe on the road.

KEEP YOUR VEHICLE IN GOOD SHAPE

Half of making sure you're safe with your vehicle is being aware and using common sense. The other half is having a backup plan in case your first line of preparation falls short. Imagine you get a flat tire. You pull over and get ready to change it, but when you open your trunk and get out the spare, you realize it is deflated, too. You might be stuck for some time while waiting for a towing service. But if you had purchased a can of tire inflator—you can get one in any automotive store—and put it in your trunk, you could have fixed the spare and made it to a gas station or tire shop on your own.

Pay heed to the warning signs your vehicle gives you before they turn into an emergency. Has your engine been making a strange noise lately? Does your car overheat a bit after idling for less than 10 minutes? Rather than nurse it along, make sure it is operating properly. Have your mechanic check it out. You don't want to be stranded on the side of the road in the middle of nowhere, which is often what happens when people put auto repairs and inspections off for too long. Even brand new cars can malfunction. Many cars nowadays will indicate what part of the engine or brake system needs attention, as they are built with a computerized "brain" of their own.

Be sure you stay in control by being proactive and ensuring your safety on the road.

PLAN AHEAD FOR LONGER TRIPS AND VACATIONS

Before taking a trip, make sure your car is in good condition. Have your local dealer or mechanic perform a maintenance check-up. A preventive tune-up could mean the difference between life or death on the road. Make sure your tires are in good condition, along with your spare (and your can of tire inflator).

Plan ahead! Ideally, you should always know ahead of time where the gas stations are located, how much fuel it will take to get from Point A to Point B, how many miles you'll be driving, how long it will take you to reach your destination, what time of day you will be driving and what the weather forecast is for the area you'll be traveling through. Start your journey with a full gas tank and fill it regularly as you travel. A good rule of thumb is: Never allow your tank to go below half. You never know when the stations in some of the small towns on your trip might shut down early, leaving you stranded. For extra preparation, especially on long distance drives through thinly populated areas, carry a spare gas can.

Keep important items such as a blanket, a few snacks and water with you at all times. Make sure your cell phone is fully charged when you're on the road. Better yet, invest in a charger that can be hooked up to your car.

Always leave as much information as you can about your trip and schedule with relatives, friends or neighbors. If anything goes wrong, they will at least know where you should be at a certain time. You also want to check in with them at regular times so they know that you are all right. If your car breaks down or has some other problem, call and let someone know where you are and what the problem is. Also, call before you get going again, so they will know you are OK.

Never pick up hitchhikers! Sure, your intentions may be good, but inviting a total stranger into your car is never a good idea. If you see someone stranded, call the police and let them handle it. That way you're not jeopardizing your safety and well-being but are still doing your part to assist someone in trouble.

Sometimes there are people standing on the side of freeways asking for money or food. Many drivers will stop, feeling sorry for them, not realizing that they could be decoys for other criminals or a gang.

In one instance, a state trooper stopped to help a motorist stranded on the side of the road. Thinking nothing of it, the officer assumed the man just needed to call a tow truck. But when he came to the hood of the truck and asked the man to step away from the front of his vehicle, the man started to shoot at him. The state trooper only stopped to help him. The good news was the officer was not seriously injured and the criminal was apprehended.

However, it doesn't always turn out so well, so be careful.

RESEARCH UNFAMILIAR AREAS

Victim prevention includes preparing ahead of time. If you're going to a place you've never been before, the best thing is to google the address and become familiar with the area from information gathered online. That is as true for other parts of the city where you live as it is for another state or country.

If friends ask you to meet them somewhere you've never been before, check ahead of time if there are any construction delays or detours along the route. Better yet, have them meet at your house or a familiar gathering point so you can all go together. That way no one gets lost or arrives late. Investigate the meeting place beforehand, including location and hours of service. I know plenty of people who have made a date to meet someone at a restaurant, only to discover that it was closed (or even out of business) when they got there, because they didn't bother to check ahead of time.

Whenever you drive to a new area, keep your car doors locked. This makes it impossible for someone to jump into your car at a stoplight, as has happened to unsuspecting travelers.

Many new cars come equipped with GPS (Global Positioning System) navigation systems such as OnStar. Even if your car doesn't have such a device, you can purchase one for when you travel to unknown areas. Many new cell phones and PDAs (Personal Digital Assistants) come with or can be set up with a GPS to get you out of trouble when you're lost. Be sure to download maps of the areas you will be traveling before you leave. You'll want the most up-to-date versions. If you bought your system two years ago and the roads have been changed due to construction, for example, your GPS may lead you on a wild and frustrating goose chase.

Find out as much as you can about the conditions on the route you'll be traveling. Are the roads OK? Are they well-lit? Try to limit your route to well-traveled roads.

WHAT TO DO IN BAD WEATHER

Check the weather report for your travel route and destination on television or online before heading out. Even so, weather can change unexpectedly. If you get caught in a bad storm and can't see in front of you while driving, you have a good chance of getting hurt. Keep your emergency flashing lights on, pull all the way off the road, and wait until the heaviest downpour passes. Listen to the local radio station. If severe weather is forecast for an extended period of time, find a hotel and stay until conditions improve. Otherwise, you could simply go to a diner or restaurant and wait out the storm. Stay at a hotel with a recognizable name and reputation. You can also look for an alternate route in order to avoid the storms if you are comfortable with the area and have a trusted GPS or map.

Rental cars

A few years ago, gangs in Miami targeted travelers who rented cars at the airport. They noted the special codes on license plates that indicated rental vehicles. The criminals would deliberately bump the cars from behind and when the unsuspecting drivers stopped, rob them. It became an international issue when a German tourist was shot and killed. Police crackdown and education alleviated the problem then, but staying alert to your surroundings is always a good idea.

Whether you're on a business trip or vacation, when you rent a car make sure you know the emergency service offered by the company. How long is the company's average response time? Is it 24-hour service? Who do you call if you need help or road assistance? Always know all pertinent information and never take for granted that there won't be a problem. When traveling in a rental car, do not drive in deserted areas where you can't get help quickly or easily. Your best bet is to take a well-lit route. If you must call for help, say you need assistance immediately. When help arrives, be sure to fully check out the person who pulls up to make sure he is with the company the rental agency mentioned. Also, use your cell phone to let your family and friends know your location in case something happens before road assistance arrives. In fact, it may be a good idea to stay on the line with your family until you are sure you're safe and secure.

If you are in an accident, follow the procedures mentioned earlier.

Conclusion

Always think ahead. If you have made good plans for safe traveling, you will have taken care of 90% of any difficulties you're likely to encounter. Beyond that, use common sense. Remember, even if you stop to have a bite to eat, always stay vigilant regarding your surroundings, and be careful how much information you give out about yourself. If someone asks where you are headed, think twice about answering. Consider giving the name of a nearby town, even if you're not headed that way.

You want to savor the pleasure of the exciting experience of traveling and looking at all the wonders new places have to offer, while avoiding difficult or dangerous situations.

5 POINT PLAN

1. Do not stop for anyone on the side of the road. Call the authorities to take care of anyone who needs help.

2. Stay inside your car with the doors locked while pumping gas at night.

3. In case of an accident, stay inside your car and call 911 before dealing with the other party involved.

4. Have your car checked out and tuned up before you go on any extended trip.

5. Check out your route and destination ahead of time in as much detail as you can gather, including road and weather conditions.

Chapter 6

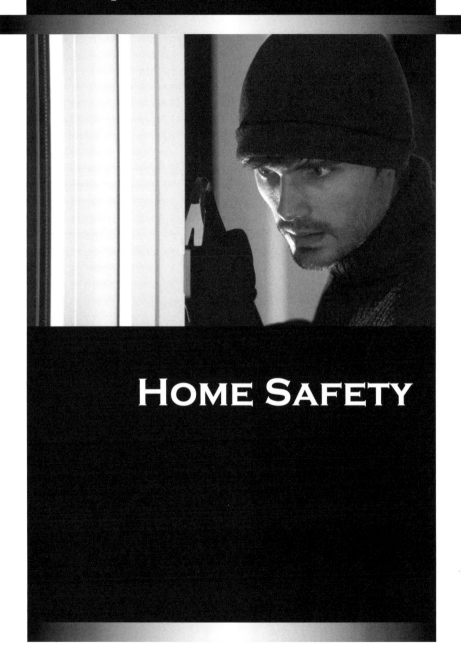

HOME SAFETY

The 17th-century English jurist Sir Edward Coke was quoted as saying, "For a man's house is his castle, *et domus sua cuique tutissimum refugium*" ("and one's home is the safest refuge for all"). It may have been true in Coke's time, and many continue to believe that it is so to this day, even though the facts don't bear them out. Turn on the evening news in most towns and cities throughout the United States, and you will see any number of stories about home invasions that make it clear that people's homes are no longer the secure refuges we would like them to be.

When it comes to safety in our own homes, there are three types of events that put us at serious risk: One is criminals committing home invasions (robberies when the inhabitants are present); another is drive-by shootings, which occur with increasing frequency in some neighborhoods, especially if they are in or near gang territory; the third is Mother Nature in the form of storms, earthquakes and other natural disasters.

HOME INVASIONS

In 1966, Truman Capote published *In Cold Blood*, a riveting account of the brutal murders of a wealthy farmer, his wife and their two children in Holcomb, Kansas, at the hands of two ex-convicts who invaded their home. The crimes took place in 1959, and the killers were caught and later executed by hanging. At the time, the book caused a sensation, not only because of the graphic account of the appalling crime, but because home invasions were not all that common, and most Americans never considered the possibility that their home might be under attack.

Those innocent times are long gone. While such crimes are always shocking, they are no longer a rarity nowadays. In fact, home invasions are on the rise, all over the country, even in gated communities where walls, fences and guards at the entrance give residents a false sense of security.

As I am writing this chapter, one of the two men who committed a particularly horrific home invasion in Cheshire, Connecticut in 2007 is undergoing trial. The case received national media attention—again in part because of the random, terrifying nature of the crime. According to the confession of the defendant, he and his partner planned only to rob the house, but "things got out of hand." So much so that they severely beat the doctor who owned the house (he was the only survivor), and sexually assaulted and killed his wife and two daughters. The two men were caught fleeing the scene after they set fire to the house to burn the evidence.

Fortunately, such dreadful cases don't happen every day, but the data regarding home invasions is anything but reassuring.

Home invasion is defined as "burglary of a dwelling while the residents are at home." Although the intruders may only break in to steal jewelry, money and expensive audio and video equipment, such as television sets and computers, the presence of the residents often leads to more serious crimes, including sexual assault, rape and murder.

There are 8,000 home invasions in North America daily! Over the course of one year, that means nearly three million homes, or one in five, experience this crime.

According to a United States Department of Justice report:

- 38% of assaults occur during home invasions. 60% of rapes occur during home invasions.
- 50% of home invasions involve the use of weapons, the most common being knives.
- 17% of home invasion victims are age 60 or older.
- 68% of home invasions are by strangers.
- 11% of home invasions are committed by friends, business associates or family members of the victim.

Perhaps the most frightening aspect of home invasions is that the criminals can often go about their business without being noticed by the neighbors, leaving the victims helpless and at the mercy of their perpetrators.

HAVE A PLAN

Imagine sitting on the couch, watching a movie with your family, when someone barges in through the front door waving a weapon, demanding to know where you keep your jewelry. Whether you have two or five seconds to react, there's never enough time to plan when you're in the middle of such a crisis.

People think they are safe because they have installed an alarm system (with signs indicating so on the front lawn), or keep guns in the house, or own a big dog. But these "safety measures" just lull them into a false sense of security. The expensive motion detection system is probably off, so it won't protect you. If the criminals peeked in through a window beforehand, they will know if you're armed. Chances are, even if you have weapons to protect you in your home, you won't have them in hand while enjoying "family movie night" on the sofa, and Fido may be in the backyard.

Yes, surprise attack is the preferred method criminals are using today. Think about it...you hear someone kicking in your door. By the time you respond to grab your phone, it'll be too late. The criminals will already be in your home and the safety of your loved ones instantly will be compromised.

Criminals consider the head of the household to be their biggest threat in most cases, so they will target him or her right away. They have no fear forcing their way into your home in the middle of the day or at night. They are bold and dangerous and have no remorse. They don't care about your property, your family or your safety. They count on the shock and surprise, and are likely to do whatever it takes to get what they want.

The best way to protect yourself from these brutal criminals is to develop an emergency plan. Rehearse it until each family member knows how to react without panic or confusion. Then, if something does happen, the element of surprise won't incapacitate you and allow the criminals to succeed. Remember, you're dealing with only a moment's notice. It can take as little as 1.7 seconds to break down a front door.

NATURAL DISASTERS

Depending on which part of the Unites States you live in, you and your home may be at risk for the following disasters: winter storms, hurricanes, tornadoes, earthquakes, mudslides, brush and forest fires, and floods, to name a few. Any of them can become devastating events that put you and your family in danger.

While there are early warning signs for some natural disasters—with hurricanes, for example, we often know as far as a week in advance about the possible paths they will take—others, like tornadoes, can strike all of a sudden. In either case, it is best to be prepared ahead of time.

Often, staying safe requires having a backup plan, in case the first plan falls through. In the event of a major storm in your area, for example, do you have more than one plan for picking up the kids from school and getting home from work? What if the roads on your regular route are flooded and streets are closed? Do you know the alternate ways to take? Have you arranged with other parents or neighbors to perhaps pick your children up instead?

What do you do if a disaster like a tornado, hurricane or flooding threatens and requires you to evacuate your home? Do you wait until the police officers come to your door and tell you to go, or do you leave ahead of time? Do you have an evacuation route planned? Do you know where you are going to stay? If you have pets, do you know which shelters will allow you to bring them with you? Have you made a list ahead of time of what valuables you should take? Do you have your legal papers in a file box that you can grab quickly, or are they already in a secure safety deposit box? Do you have your computer backed up to a portable hard drive or via the Internet?

It is very important to have a plan for all of these things before disaster strikes. If you have to think about these things when the crisis hits, along with keeping your family safe, it can be too much to handle.

PLANS AND PREPARATIONS

One of the most important things we can do—whether we are the man or the woman of the house, in a couple or as a single parent—is to understand what it takes to keep our families safe. We need to be in a proactive mode and have plans in place, so we're not just reacting when something happens. Preparedness is the best way to counter the element of surprise. We also need to teach our children and loved ones how to take action. They must receive training to be aware of what can happen around them and know exactly what to do in the event a bad situation occurs.

HOUSE RULES

There should be a set of house rules for everyone to follow in the event of a traumatic situation (such as a natural disaster, a fire, or home invasion). All family members should know which door or window to use in case they need to get out of the house quickly. A two- or three-story house should have an emergency rope ladder that can be used to exit from the upper stories, and everyone should know how to deploy it.

There should always be someone in charge, preferably a parent or an older member of the family who understands what is happening and knows what to do. At the same time, there should be a clear understanding of everyone's responsibilities—what each family member can be expected to do—including the children, no exceptions.

When it comes to sudden natural events, such as tornadoes or an earthquake, everyone in the family should know exactly where to go to be safe. It could be the hallway outside their rooms, a closet in the center of the house, the bathroom on the first floor, or the basement. Family members caught on upper floors should get down to ground level if at all possible. The older children should know which one of the younger children they are responsible for in a dangerous situation. Maintaining a head count and knowing that everyone is safe will offer some comfort.

In the case of a home invasion, the family should know which room has a strong lock and can be used as a safe room, and go there as quickly as possible.

STRENGTHEN DOORS

Besides developing a plan for a home invasion, there are some concrete things you can do in advance of it actually happening. The most vulnerable spot of your house is the front door (or in some cases, the back door—houses that have French doors opening onto a lanai or backyard are especially vulnerable). To protect yourself, you need a real barrier, something that doesn't splinter in a matter of seconds. Invest in a solid wood or metal door and equip it with a strong lock. A sturdy door and heavy-duty lock are like the medieval portcullis, the iron grill that was lowered inside the castle gate to fend off enemy attack. There are doors and locks on the market that will keep the assailants occupied and even frustrate them to the point where they might give up. One such lock on the market withstands up to 4,000 pounds of force. Even a police battering ram has a hard time defeating it. (For more information, see the Appendix.)

Think: Is it worth the extra money to install a heavier and more solid door in your home's entrance areas? At the least, it will buy you and your family extra time to react and execute your safety plan. Remember, you want to make it as hard as possible for criminals to break in.

You're probably asking, "If such a lock exists, why should I prepare for anything?" The truth is, the lock's main purpose is not to keep the criminals out completely, but to buy you time. There may still be danger ahead in the event the criminals have other means of trying to get in or plan to set fire to the house. However, their initial attempt and failure (due to the lock system) give you the opportunity to get your family to safety, call the authorities, and let them respond. Criminals know that they have limited time to accomplish what they want. Confronted with a powerful obstacle, they'll understand that they're dealing with someone who is prepared and may leave instead of hanging around until they hear the police sirens.

CREATE A SAFE ROOM

To really be prepared against home invasion, you need to have a place for survival, a safe room. Examine your home and designate a location where you and your family members can go and be protected if a crisis occurs. It doesn't have to be a high-tech or fancy "panic room," as in the Jodie Foster movie of the same name. It could be a bedroom, a den or the basement. The doors to this room should be solid wood, not hollow core, and the locks should be as powerful as the one on the front door, withstanding up to 4,000 pounds of force.

Make sure you have essential resources and supplies in your survival location. There should be a working cell phone in the room that is fully charged so you can call 911 or the police (landlines can be cut). Even an old cell phone that is no longer on a service plan will work. Once you power it up, you can call 911 with it. Not many people know this, and little details like that can mean the difference between life and death.

In case the criminals cut the electric power to your home, have flashlights and candles ready. If you have weapons in your home, this is the place to store them—in a safe, but easily accessible spot. Also, make sure there is a way to get out of that room through a window or door, if necessary.

When calling 911, stay as calm as possible, speak clearly and give a description of the criminals. The last thing you want to do is delay the response because the operator can't understand what you're saying. Try to keep your emotions in check, even if the situation feels desperate. Fortunately, many people act with composure until they know they are out of danger, when it is safe to break down emotionally.

REHEARSE YOUR PLAN

Just as schools and large businesses post maps of exit routes and conduct fire drills from time to time, so that people know what to do and where to go in case of a real crisis, you should "role play" various scenarios with your family. Make sure that they can quickly answer if you ask them, "When you need to get out of the house, where should you go?" Tell them they must not move until they know for sure that the coast is clear, before they run to get help. Instruct them that once they have reached the safe room in your house, to wait until the authorities get there and not to attempt "hero work" in the meantime.

Make a game out of role playing for younger children. One of the parents can be the "bad guy" in different situations and see how everyone applies the rules that have been established. Be sure all family members understand the consequences of what could happen in a real situation if they do not follow them. Use real life examples from the newspapers and TV news to explain what could happen.

Create plans for a house fire, a break-in while you are in the house, coming home to find the house has been broken into, someone getting hurt at home, and other possibilities. Walk through the steps you want your family to take for each scenario.

Talk about the requirements for the plans to be successful. For example, in case of a power outage, everyone should know where the flashlights and candles are stored. If the plan requires a backup food supply, everyone should know where to access it. All family members should also know the basics about how to treat wounds in case of an injury. Most importantly, ALL family members should know when and why calling 911 is vital to your safety.

Practice and do the drills from time to time. I can tell you from my years of law enforcement experience, that in police training everything is practiced over and over again until it becomes a routine. That way we can react without having to think about it. In fact, in 90% of actual situations, we're reacting to something we have practiced beforehand!

When you have a fire drill or practice a home invasion response, compliment the members of your family on proper execution of the plan. Say something like, "We did well. Everything is in place, and everyone went to the areas they were supposed to go to. Our plan worked." This will help you and your family gain self-esteem and confidence, which in turn will help you all to handle situations faster and more smoothly if they actually occur.

DRIVE-BY SHOOTINGS

If you live in an area where drive-by crimes are not only possible, but common, you may be worried about your personal safety and the safety of your family. It's a terrible feeling to realize you may not be safe, even in your own home. Sure, you can buy various locking devices, never answer the door to strangers and keep your kids safely playing indoors. But, in the case of a drive-by shooting, none of these measures matter. You can live in a high-security home and still be a victim. However, there are things you can do to keep yourself safe.

If you're afraid that stray bullets may come flying into your home, you should keep furniture in front of your windows as a buffer against any possible shootings. You may want to set up your house or apartment in such a way that the areas where the family spends a great deal of time, including watching television and sleeping, are in the rear. That way, walls and doors can become natural barriers. You can install bulletproof windows if you can afford them. At least make sure your front door is constructed of high-quality materials, like hard wood or metal, so that they can resist bullets fired in the direction of your home.

It is also important for you to learn CPR and how to dress a wound, in case someone is injured in your home. That way you can help yourself and your family members until the authorities and EMS squad arrive.

These safety tips may seem over the top, but if you happen to live in a neighborhood next to gang territory, taking these precautions may save your life.

FRONT YARD SAFETY

If you live in an area where drive-by shootings are common, it's never a good idea to let your children play in the front yard or on the front porch. However, if you do want to let your kids enjoy the outdoors, never allow them to do so unsupervised. You, or someone you trust, should be on the lookout for signs of potential trouble. Chances are, you know the people who are associated with gang activity. If you see their car coming around the corner, quickly get your kids inside. If you notice an unfamiliar car coming down the street (in a normally un-trafficked neightborhood), move to safety. Being aware of your surroundings can help you keep your family safe.

It is also crucial that you teach your children what to do if they hear shots or suspect that a drive-by shooting might occur. Instead of standing up and running inside (or worse, waiting to watch what will happen), they should hit the ground on their stomachs and not move. It's what soldiers do under fire, and your children will be, if only for a moment, in a combat zone. Once they're confident that the car is gone, they can then crawl on their stomachs to safety. Practice drills with them, so they know what to expect and what to do to stay safe.

INSIDE THE HOUSE

If a drive-by shooting occurs while you are in your home, immediately get as low as possible. Lie on the floor on your stomach and cover small children with your body. Drive-by shootings typically last a few seconds. So when you notice the shots have stopped, crawl to the rear of the house and call 911. If you can peek out the window safely, check to see what color and make the shooter's car is and the direction it is heading to give to the police when they arrive. Don't exit your home! Be sure to wait until the authorities have cleared the area and given you permission to do so.

STRANGERS AT THE DOOR

Just as important as being prepared against forcible home invasion or drive-by shootings is being ready to deal with more subtle assaults. One of the hardest things criminals have to deal with is getting inside a house without alerting others in the neighborhood. Crashing through a front door can be a noisy affair that draws undue attention. As a result, some of them have become creative in how to get inside a house in other ways, especially when they know there are children at home alone. They may pose as meter readers, deliverymen, or people selling cookies and other products in the neighborhood.

Make sure children understand that if a stranger knocks, they may not answer the door—no matter what the circumstances! Explain to them that it is not necessary to open the door to see who is there. They can look out of a window or ask through the door to find out. If they do not recognize the person, under no circumstances should they open the door! Instead, they should ask the person to come back later. Have them mention that their parents will be home any moment. If adults are in the house, children should let them know that someone is at the door and have an adult open the door.

If a deliveryman comes to the door with a package and claims he needs it to be signed for, have children who are home alone request that he leave a note in the mailbox indicating where the item can be picked up later.

You yourself have the right to ask for identification before opening the door to any deliveryman. FedEx or UPS drivers come in a truck with the corporate logo on the side and all have ID from their respective companies, usually attached to the front pocket of their shirt. The truck should be parked at the curb in plain view, not somewhere around the corner. The drivers will also carry computerized consoles for you to sign if they require a signature. If no signature is required, they will leave the package on the porch or by the door.

Bottom line: No one should answer the door without an adult present.

LATCHKEY KIDS

Following these safety measures is especially important for latchkey kids, who come home in the afternoon and spend some hours alone before their parents get off from work. Sometimes they bring schoolmates along to play or do homework together. Be sure that your children's friends, too, understand your house rules and the reasons for them, and are prepared to follow them to the letter.

Explain to them that you are not being mean, but you want to make sure they can live and play in a secure environment. The parents of your children's friends should be grateful to you for trying to keep everyone in safe surroundings while they are in your home.

CARETAKERS AND SITTERS

Similarly, it is important that those who look after your children in your absence, such as babysitters, nannies and other caretakers, know what the house rules are. They should not open the door to anyone they have not been told to expect. Your children and the sitter should be instructed that if someone becomes overly aggressive trying to get inside the house, they are to call you on your cell phone immediately. If they cannot reach you, they should call the police or 911. If they do reach you and you do not feel right about the situation, call the police yourself and let them deal with the problem.

EXERCISE LEADERSHIP

The head of the household, whether in a single-parent or two-parent family, is the one who brings confidence to the home. It is very important for him or her to maintain a level of self-assurance that he or she can make the right decisions when necessary. In a two-parent family, usually the mother is more involved with watching out for the safety of the children than the father. If she feels uncomfortable about a particular situation, she should keep her cell phone handy with the speed dial set to 911.

STAY IN TOUCH

Everyone in the family should know the schedules of all the other family members—when they are coming and going, and where they will be when not at home. Have everyone check in when they arrive at a destination, when they are leaving to come home or when they head to another location. This makes it possible to keep track of everyone and respond quickly if something unforeseen happens. With the convenience of cell phones and text messaging, there should be no reason to be out of touch for long.

If you do not hear from someone as expected, contact them to make sure everything is OK. Perhaps there was an accident or heavy traffic, which has delayed them from coming home at the appointed time. Also, keeping in frequent communication lets children know you are concerned about them and that they need to stick to a schedule so you will know they are safe.

Be sure to get to know your children's teachers and communicate with them often. We are very busy with the demands of living today, but that should not prevent us from contacting teachers to make sure our children are doing well in school, and that there are no problems that might endanger them either at school or on the way home. Technology has given us e-mail as well as cell phones to make it easier to stay in touch. Teachers like to know that parents are interested in their children's progress at school, and are more likely to let you know about any problems that could affect the safety of your children if they know you care.

KEEP INFORMED

I have mentioned this before, but it bears repeating. Always check for crime and problems happening in your community by reading your local newspapers, going to neighborhood and homeowners' association meetings, participating in your local PTA, and listening to TV and radio news programs. If problems occur repeatedly in your area, inform your local police and even let the newspapers and media know about it. Perhaps they will report it, which will let others know what is happening. News coverage can also lead to the police becoming more active in your area. This alone could make it safer for you and your family.

Show and explain what you see and hear to your family, so they understand that the rules and plans you have put in place have a real purpose for helping to keep the family safe. Knowledge is power, and the more knowledge your family members have about what is going on around them, the more power they will have to cope with problems if they arise.

CALL ON NEIGHBORHOOD SUPPORT

It's a great idea for your neighborhood to develop code words to use in crisis situations. Sometimes, when a criminal breaks into a home and a neighbor notices something odd going on, he or she will knock on the door, asking if there's a problem. Criminals know that if they don't allow you to answer, the neighbor might call the police right away. Therefore, they will demand that you say there's nothing wrong, usually without opening the door (just yelling your response). If your neighborhood has a secret code phrase for crisis situations like "I'll call you tomorrow," it will alert your neighbor that something is wrong, without the criminal catching on. You can choose a single word or phrase, but be sure it sounds natural in conversation, so the criminal won't be alerted.

CONCLUSION

Remember, doors and alarm systems can help keep you safe, but ultimately, being prepared is your best form of protection. With the combination of alarm systems, high-security door locks, a safe room, a neighborhood watch, a good plan in case of natural disasters or home invasions, and overall vigilance and awareness, there is hope to once again feel as safe in your home as if it were a castle!

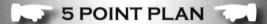

5 POINT PLAN

1. Have a well-rehearsed plan in place for all emergencies, including home invasions, drive-by shootings and natural disasters.

2. Arm all entrances to your home with solid doors and high-quality locks.

3. Create a safe room inside the house where you and your family can go in case of a home invasion.

4. Make sure your children know what to do regarding strangers at the door when they are home alone.

5. Stay in touch with family members throughout the day.

Chapter 7

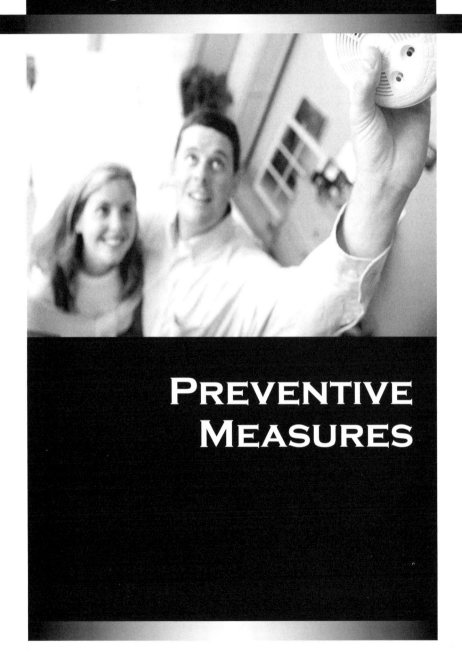

PREVENTIVE MEASURES

So what can you do to protect yourself against the potential dangers at home, at work and at play? This chapter will discuss a number of options. You may wish to pursue some or all of them. There will be some overlap with solutions proposed in previous chapters— but looking at them from another perspective may prove helpful and allow you to understand their importance better. Remember, the goal is not 100% safety and security—that is impossible—but to give you an edge and buy you time. Also remember that criminals prefer the course of least resistance, so letting them know in one way or another that you will not be an easy victim is likely to give them pause and encourage them to look elsewhere.

Above all, know that you can do many things to reduce your personal vulnerability and take measures to protect yourself and those you love. The better you are prepared, the more you will feel in control of your life.

KEEP YOUR DOORS LOCKED

Always keep your front and back doors locked. You've likely heard this a million times, but safety is all about making it harder for the criminal to execute a crime. You would be amazed at how many people leave the front door to their house open while they are getting groceries out of the car. As they bend over to lift the bags from the trunk or backseat, criminals can slip inside unobserved and wait for them there. Sometimes something as simple as locking the door can save your life.

HAVE EMERGENCY NUMBERS HANDY

Keep emergency numbers in as many places as possible—in the house, in your car, and in your wallet or purse. These include phone numbers for the police, fire department, doctors, family members, neighbors and friends. Keep a list of emergency numbers on your refrigerator. Also, be sure to program all emergency numbers into your cell phone, so you can get to them quickly when needed.

DEAL QUICKLY WITH LOST KEYS

Many parents worry about their children losing their house keys, but it happens to many adults as well. In either case, it's vital to take swift action. If there is no hope of finding the keys quickly, you must have the locks changed immediately—the sooner they are, the less likely you are to become a victim of a home invasion.

Criminals watch and wait in parking lots, on the bus or in the subway, for you to drop your keys. They may even quietly snatch them while you're not looking. They then follow you home and wait for you and your family to go to bed. When they feel the "coast is clear," they use the keys to enter your home.

If you live in an apartment or a college dorm and you lose your key, it's important to notify management immediately. Be firm and insist that your locks get changed that same day. After all, your safety is on the line! If management refuses to comply with your request, stay with a friend or family member, or in a hotel, until the locks are changed.

EXPLAIN SAFETY RULES TO YOUR CHILDREN

If you want to ensure that your children know how to stay safe, you must explain to them the need to be alert and aware. Don't assume that they understand the issues involved. It is vital that you teach them specific actions and safety techniques. Make sure they know what's going on in the neighborhood and around school. You don't want to unnecessarily scare your children, but you also don't want them to let their guard down. It's much like teaching them not to cross the street unless a crossing guard is present or they are with an adult. Likewise, your children should know what to do in other potentially dangerous situations.

VARY ROUTINES

All human beings are creatures of habit. We put on clothes in the same order every morning. We leave for work at the same time each day and we turn the lights off to go to bed around the same time each night. But, have you ever thought that someone might be watching you and taking note that you leave at 9:00 a.m. every morning to take little Johnny to school? Or that you return around 10:15 and leave again at noon to go to the bank, and always come back for lunch at 1:30 p.m.?

Criminals often stake out a family before making their move to determine when to attack, so they have the best chance to be in control. They may force their way in when they know a teenager is the only person in the house, or when a stay-at-home mom has just dropped her children off at school. Most criminals assume that the man of the house is the most dangerous family member and are not as likely to invade if they know he is at home.

To deter criminals from memorizing your schedule, vary your routine throughout the week. Be unpredictable. Go to the grocery store at random hours, instead of every Monday morning at 10:00 a.m. like clockwork. Leave for work a few minutes earlier than usual some mornings. Travel to and from work by different routes and, if possible, keep changing how long you are gone from home. That way you will throw a wrench into their preferred way of operating.

BE ALERT AROUND MONEY

One time to be extra careful is upon exiting the bank. Perhaps it's Friday and you've just cashed your paycheck. Criminals may be staking out people like you, counting on you to have a pocket full of money. They can target you quickly and attack even before you get to your car. Never draw attention to yourself by flashing cash in public. Money is a private matter and should be kept out of public view.

Do not take unnecessary risks

When you're 16 and the kid next door dares you to eat an extra hot jalapeño, chances are you'll rise to the occasion and take the risk (and suffer the consequences). After all, as a teenager, you're likely to feel that you have something to prove. But as an adult in today's world, being a risk taker when it comes to your safety and that of your family's is never a good idea. If you encounter a dangerous situation, stay in a place where you can observe what is going on, but don't interfere and put your life on the line. That is the job of the authorities. They are professionals trained to handle such matters. Give them a call instead of trying to save the day on your own.

On the other hand, you don't have to be passive. Let's say you are driving and come upon a gang beating someone. You need to be able to react quickly and call the authorities. But it will also help later on if you can provide a clear description of the attackers, including the size of the individuals involved (big, fat, thin, small, tall), their ages (teenagers, mid-20s), what clothes they are wearing (jeans, sweatshirts, hoodies) and in what colors (blue, black, tan, with designs or pictures), as well as any visible scars or tattoos. Although things can happen very fast, try to be ready to provide the police with as much information as possible so the attackers can be apprehended. Remember, at some point it could be your family or loved ones you save with the information you supply to the police. Your attention to details, which comes with practice and training your mind to notice them, could save someone you love!

Avoid being alone

Are you a solitary person? Do you like to spend time by yourself? Do you frequently go out alone? I don't want to cramp your lifestyle, but to stay safe, it's best to travel in pairs or groups.

Remember, there's safety in numbers. If you have a close friend, try to plan outings like grocery shopping, going to the hairdresser or visiting the mall when you can do them together. You're much less vulnerable when traveling with another person than if you are alone. Think about it...even police officers go on their shifts in pairs whenever possible.

JOIN A NEIGHBORHOOD WATCH

I can tell you that law enforcement professionals are very encouraged to see more and more people participating in community crime awareness programs. As they say, "Four eyes see better than two," and a well-organized watch group will notice even more and deter criminals by its very presence. There are now several types of active groups, such as Citizens On Patrol, that raise the standard of safety by their attentiveness to what is happening in the local neighborhoods, schools and businesses.

If there is such an organization patrolling your neighborhood, consider joining. Participating will make you more aware of what is happening in your community and allow you to contribute to everyone's safety. It also gives you an opportunity to become acquainted with your local law enforcement officers who patrol the area. Police officers want you to know that they are active in your area. They also want you to feel comfortable asking questions and informing them as soon as you notice something unusual that should be looked into. Something as simple as letting them know what you have seen on patrol might keep a problem from developing, because they know what to watch for.

FREQUENT OTHER COMMUNITY ORGANIZATIONS

At a time when there is an increasing shortage of police officers in many departments throughout the country, local citizens getting involved is a key element to fighting crime. Consider holding town hall meetings to discuss what's happening in your neighborhood. Invite local authorities and elected officials. These meetings are excellent opportunities to voice concerns and discuss odd goings-on, such as strangers driving around your neighborhood for no apparent reason.

If you're unable to hold town hall meetings, organize your neighbors. You can collect their complaints and send them via e-mail or by certified letter to your local elected officials. Tell them what your problems are and ask if they can help. If you put your elected officials on the spot, they will feel pressured to get results.

Attend meetings of homeowners' associations (HOAs) or property owners' associations (POAs) and make suggestions on improving security in the area. In a neighborhood of 200 or 300 houses, there are surely enough people for someone to be on watch at all times of day or night throughout the week. Exchange ideas and concepts with others and unite around the common goal of keeping your neighborhood safe. Consider organizing a block party so you can meet and greet each other and learn who is willing to be a part of the watch patrol.

The presence of retirees in a neighborhood is often helpful. Many enjoy being involved in something important that benefits others as well as themselves. Let them voice their opinions and listen to what they have to say. They can be a strong element of support, and because they tend not to sleep as long as younger people, they may notice things at night that those who watch in the early morning hours and throughout the day might miss.

Community awareness courses held by the police are another great way to stay informed in regard to crimes and other safety concerns that affect your community. Knowing what is going on in your children's schools, for example—from the breakout of a serious illness to a disgruntled bus driver—will allow you to be prepared to deal with any fallout.

MAKE YOUR HOME SAFE

Many people question the safety of their home. They wonder if their doors are strong enough, if they need a window alarm system or if they should install more exterior lighting. However, there are many other factors at play. For instance, home safety measures can vary depending on whether you live in a house or an apartment. Traditionally, houses are more secure. That is because apartments are usually accessible to others when the tenant is not at home. Handymen, apartment managers and landlords often have keys, putting the renter potentially at risk. It's all too easy to duplicate a key. In many apartment buildings, managers don't even change locks when tenants move out. This means a former resident may still have a key to your place. It's a good idea to talk with your landlord and insist on changing the locks.

Ten years ago, it was almost unheard of for a burglar to enter a home if he knew that the family was sleeping inside. In fact, criminals almost always planned their home break-ins at times when the family was at work, in school or on vacation. However, criminals are getting increasingly desperate, and they now break into homes while the families are sleeping, or even when still awake. They thrive on the element of surprise and figure they will have the upper hand if they attack when the family least expects it.

INSTALL AN ALARM SYSTEM

The first line of defense is to install a good alarm system, not only for when your family is away, but for when you are at home as well. Many homeowners avoid taking such precautionary security measures because they feel alarms don't work, but that kind of thinking is not based on actual knowledge. In fact, alarms not only notify you of an unwanted entry, but they serve another purpose, too. Often, when criminals break into a home and hear the alarm go off, they will retreat and leave. They know the family has been alerted, and the security company is notifying the police, ruining the element of surprise.

A good security system can cost around $360 per year, and besides offering protection, can also save you money on your home-owner's insurance. When you buy a new home, the first question insurance companies usually ask is whether or not you have a security system installed. If you do, they will give you monthly insurance discounts, saving you money over time.

Different alarm systems come with different benefits. Some monitored systems will notify the police directly or through the security company if your alarm goes off, resulting in the authorities getting dispatched immediately to check things out. Less expensive systems may only warn you of an intruder but won't notify police. Thus it is very important for you to understand the purpose and benefits of your particular alarm system, so you can modify your safety plan according to its capabilities. For instance, you may have to physically call 911 when your alarm goes off to alert the authorities.

There is another important aspect to consider. Many households have motion detection security systems, which are only enabled if the family is away from home or in bed at night. They don't protect you at other times. Even with security systems that operate during waking hours, many families forget to enable them while they are at home, relaxing.

Please remember that the point of alarms is to alert, not to protect; you will need a stronger barrier for that. But I certainly recommend including an alarm system in your arsenal of defense.

ARM YOUR COLLEGE DORMS

For those living in dorms or other residential places where alarms aren't permitted, there are other forms of protection available. Door-stop alarms, for example, can be purchased for relatively little money. Placed under the dorm room door, these alarms create a frightful, high-pitched noise if the door is opened from the outside. This is a great way of alerting you to intruders and giving them an unpleasant surprise. But understand that while these alarms often will scare off intruders, they may not keep them out. You must still be prepared to take action.

DON'T RELY ON GUARD DOGS OR WEAPONS

I love pets, but I don't recommend them as part of your defense system. Unless they're trained as guard dogs, you can't necessarily count on them to protect your home. Criminals have been known to shoot or even poison them, and until your pet is tested in an actual crisis, you won't know how he will react to an intruder. In the meantime, his presence may lull you into a false sense of security.

Similarly, while I fully support the right of people to protect themselves with weapons, I can recommend their use only with a strong caveat. I am familiar with enough cases in which a gun in the house failed to protect the owners, or ended up causing more harm than good. You must be well-trained in the use of your weapon and have thought through where you keep it in order for it to help protect you. (See the next chapter on specifics.) Few people have their gun lying next to them on the couch while they watch television. Given the quickness with which criminals can enter your home, it is unlikely that you will have time to go for your gun before you're incapacitated. So don't assume that owning a gun will solve any problem you might have, and don't become complacent.

For these reasons, I recommend paying more attention to defensive measures first.

INSTALL SPECIAL LOCKS AND SAFE ROOMS

Think of home safety this way: Alarms are installed to alert someone of a problem and doors are installed to form a protective barrier. Thus, in addition to house alarm systems, families should pay special attention to the quality and strength of their entry doors. Nowadays, criminals don't have the patience to pick a lock or the skill to break in without physical force, and felonies in which they simply kick in front or back doors to invade a home are on the rise. Few criminals today are "professionals," and they are only interested in making a quick score.

Countering this situation requires a two-pronged attack. First, you need to make sure your front and back doors are made of solid wood or metal. Then you need to install a high-quality security lock that can withstand up to 4,000 pounds of pressure, ensuring that even the strongest criminal will be unable to kick the door in. Such locks can also turn any bedroom, bathroom or basement into a "safe room," where you and your family can go in case of trouble. (See Appendix for information on The Ultimate Lock.)

CONCLUSION

With the combination of alarms, high-security door locks, neighborhood patrols, overall awareness, and a good, well-rehearsed safety plan, you are in excellent shape for whatever may happen. I can't say it enough: Being prepared for anything is your best form of protection.

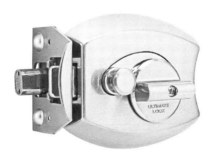

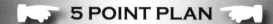

5 POINT PLAN

1. Keep emergency numbers handy at home, in your car and in your purse.

2. Do not take unnecessary risks.

3. Install an alarm system as part of your defense strategy.

4. Do not rely on dogs and weapons as your primary means of defense.

5. Make the entrances to your home safe with solid doors and high-quality locks.

Chapter 8

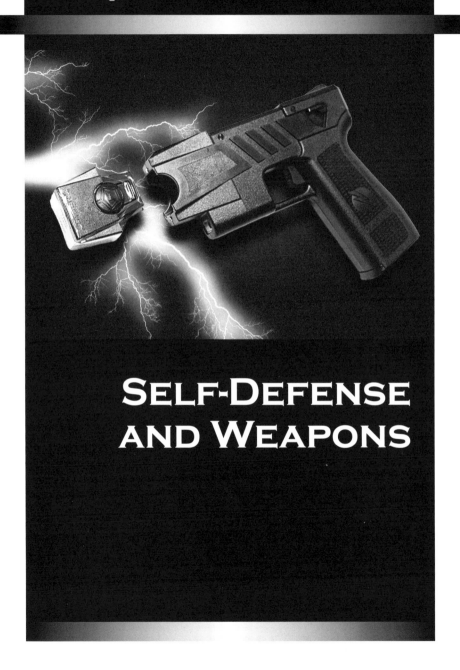

SELF-DEFENSE AND WEAPONS

Do you work out to maintain good health and look great in a bathing suit? If so, you may reap additional benefits. Being physically fit may help you in a dangerous situation. Your strength, stamina and ability will allow you to outrun potential assailants.

FIND A GOOD GYM

When searching for a good gym, look for one where you feel comfortable. That includes personnel, locker rooms, shower facilities, swimming pools and equipment. Most gyms offer a week-long trial membership. Some have separate areas where women can work out without having to worry about men ogling them. Distance from your home or place of work is important, too. Studies have shown that those who have to drive more than 20 minutes to the gym tend to let their plans to work out fall by the wayside as quickly as most other New Year's resolutions.

Along with getting fit and staying in shape, consider taking self-defense classes. To ensure you know how to react in emergencies, you need a controlled environment where you can learn what to do in specific situations. There are many places offering such courses. Do some research and make sure you find one that offers what you are looking for.

Classes may be held at the gym where you work out. Although martial arts is considered a sport, many academies offer some classes specifically geared toward self-defense, too. Check with your local police department to find out if it offers such courses; even if it doesn't, someone there can probably direct you where to find them.

When visiting venues that offer self-defense classes, ask about their success stories, how long they've been in existence, what scenarios they reenact, if they work with victims of major crimes, and if the course will build self-confidence. Ask them to tell you how they rank with other programs in town. Make clear that you want to take your ability to protect yourself to a higher level. Discuss the price of the program and the amount of time it will take to meet the standards you're trying to attain. Take only courses you feel you need. Finally, before you enroll, call their references and speak with students who have taken the courses in the past.

Remember, it is not all about the cost of the program; it's about the quality of the instruction. For example, in law enforcement we have access to different types of shooting ranges. One might be more expensive than another, but if it provides the kind of instruction that gives police officers a better edge on the streets, it's worth the extra dollars.

ADJUST YOUR MENTAL ATTITUDE

As any good self-defense instructor will tell you, more than half the battle is mental attitude. Not only will you become comfortable with certain techniques—escaping holds, immobilizing your opponent, attack and counter-attack—you will also find out how to prepare yourself. Above all, you will extend the limits of what you thought you could do.

For example, a good way to turn your fist into a more dangerous weapon is to take your house keys and hold them so that at least one key projects between your index and middle finger. But will you be ready to use it to inflict maximum damage on an assailant? Would you hesitate to poke him in the throat, or better yet, in one of his eyes? Unless you work through some of these scenarios ahead of time, you won't be ready should the occasion arise.

Ultimately, staying safe is all about taking control in emergency situations. You want to learn how to do that by gaining skills that will add to your personal confidence level. Confidence is a big word in safety. If you doubt your abilities, you may not be able to keep yourself and your family safe during emergencies. Part of building confidence is learning what to do and when to do it. It's essential that both your body and your mind are ready to snap into action and survival mode. You need to train them both how to react to situations you don't normally encounter and be ready to take extraordinary measures in extraordinary circumstances.

CONSIDER MACE, PEPPER SPRAY OR TASERS

If you are not prepared to carry a weapon, you might want to consider alternatives such as mace, pepper spray or a taser. All three can incapacitate an assailant and give you enough time to get to safety. As with guns, it is important that you practice using them ahead of time, so you can act in the heat of the moment without deliberation.

Pepper spray and mace come in pressurized cans and shoot a mist into the air that causes a burning sensation in the eyes, nose and sinuses. When receiving a full blast in the face, it becomes nearly impossible for a person to do anything but deal with the mucus, tearing and coughing. Such sprays are legal when applied strictly for self-defense, but using them in any other manner could land you in hot water with the authorities.

If you use either of these measures against an assailant, be careful. The person will be very agitated and may react by pointing a knife or discharging a gun in your direction during the few seconds before the full effect of the spray kicks in. Then, if they got a full dose in the face, they will be out of control, screaming, crying, coughing and gasping for breath. In any case, don't stick around; get yourself to safety. You also should know that distance and wind conditions can reduce the full effect. Indeed, if the wind pushes some of the spray in your face, you will experience similar results as your assailant, and feeling incapacitated and panicky will make you much more vulnerable.

When it comes to tasers, some states limit their use only to law enforcement officials. Check what laws apply in your state before carrying one. Be aware that for a taser to work, you have to be even closer than with mace or pepper spray, unless your model shoots out electrified darts into the clothing and body of your assailant.

If you miss with either sprays or tasers, however, you are likely to make your attacker angry, so I caution you once again to take a training class before carrying any of these items.

SHOULD I OWN A HANDGUN?

As with self-defense classes, whether or not to purchase a weapon is a personal matter. The danger is that some people think just owning a gun increases their safety. A young woman I know who went to a large state university felt unsafe at night in her off-campus apartment and bought a handgun, which she kept in the drawer of her bedside table. Having the weapon there reassured her, but I'd argue that she actually would be less safe if something were to happen. It goes back to planning, preparation and practice. Unless you are comfortable using a weapon like a handgun as if it were an extension of your arm, it can become a liability if you encounter a criminal who is more familiar with it than you. If he takes it away from you, it will increase the danger to you exponentially.

So if you choose to arm yourself, make sure you know how to use your weapon. Whether you have it somewhere in your home or are carrying it under a concealed weapon license (CWL), you must practice drawing it frequently until it becomes second nature. I also recommend going to a shooting range at least two to three times a month and shooting at least 50 rounds each time. Practice shooting with both hands, with your regular shooting arm, and in different stances: You never know how you might need to use your weapon.

But be aware that you're aiming at a paper target that is holding still and not shooting back; you can take your time in a relaxed environment. You don't know how you will respond in a real crisis until it happens—so it's best to be prepared for any situation.

There are a lot of other issues you may not be thinking about. For example, your gun may jam. If it's the first time, you won't know what to do and might panic. Better it should happen on the shooting range, where you can find out if it was because you did something wrong or because you had bad ammunition, rather than when you are in danger.

Let me tell you about a case in which someone who had a license to carry a gun did all the right things to protect his family, given the circumstances.

When Chet arrived home from work late one afternoon, his wife's car was in the driveway, but when he knocked on the front door, there was no answer. Something felt odd to him, so he got in his car, drove down the street and parked out of sight of his house. He returned through the backyards and carefully looked in through the windows. In the living room he saw his wife duct taped to a chair and being threatened by two intruders. One was holding a gun to her head while the other yelled questions, apparently trying to get her to tell him where money was stashed.

Since Chet had a concealed weapon license, he always carried his gun with him. He managed to crawl into the house through an open bathroom window, sneak to the living room and wait until the men took a moment to step away from his wife. Then he shot them both, killing them.

While we encourage "citizens" to call the police rather than take the law into their own hands, we felt, when we arrived and investigated, that in this case Chet's actions were justified. With the intruders brandishing their own weapons, who knows what might have happened if they had heard police sirens approaching. If they had panicked, they might have shot Chet's wife.

Two other important points: Chet was a retired Green Beret with extensive training and experience in the use of weapons. Second, he had time and the element of surprise on his side. He could methodically think through what he was going to do ahead of time, rather than have to think on his feet in the heat of the moment, and then proceed with his plan.

Most first-time gun owners have neither the experience nor the coolness under fire to use their weapons this way. So you should think very hard about whether or not having a gun would really make you safer before you rely on it for protection. If you decide to go ahead, consider the following:

Getting a weapons license

An applicant must be qualified to purchase a handgun under federal laws and the laws of a particular state that set out the eligibility criteria. Gun laws in the United States vary from state to state and are independent of, but not contradictory to, existing federal firearms laws. For example, in Texas the law states, "...anyone over the age of 18, without any felony convictions, is allowed to apply for a CWL." In many states, the Department of Motor Vehicles (DMV) regulates the licenses for concealed weapons.

There are a number of factors that may make a person temporarily or permanently ineligible to obtain a license. They include felony convictions (permanently) and Class A or B misdemeanors (five years). In cases of domestic violence, individuals are not allowed to purchase a weapon or carry a permit for one. People who suffer from a mental illness are not qualified to carry a gun.

Before applying for a license and obtaining a handgun, you must take a course, which can take between 24 to 72 hours, depending on the class. The instructors will give you a formal training session first and then schedule you for the required proficiency exam, which is a shooting exercise. If you cannot pass the proficiency test, you will not be issued a permit. Once you have completed the target training and are able to qualify, you must take a written test for your license. In most states, you'll also need to go to the police department to get fingerprinted. There is a waiting period before you can qualify for the permit. The entire process can take as little as three days or as long as six months, depending on the requirements of your home state.

Your CWL will come with an expiration date, so you'll know when you have to renew it. Again, depending on your state, a CWL could last from two to four years.

Be aware that you must follow the rules and guidelines regarding concealed weapons. If you don't, you can lose your license.

DENIED FOR YOUR CWL?

If you were denied, you can fix the problem and try again. You need to reschedule with the instructor to take the shooting range test or the written test again, depending on which you failed. If it is the former, you will have to pay for the ammunition. If it is the latter, the instructor will review the points with you, so you will be prepared when you try again. Once you have passed both tests, you are eligible under the guidelines of your state.

ISSUES TO CONSIDER

Before starting the process to get your handgun, you need to understand the major responsibility that comes with obtaining a CWL. For example, if you're in a position where you can protect someone and prevent them from being hurt before the police arrive, then you can detain the criminal. I strongly recommend you read and understand all of the rules and requirements that go with carrying a weapon before you even consider taking the required actions for a license.

You should also be aware of locations where you are not allowed to carry a weapon, even with a license. These places include hospitals, sporting events, airports, schools and any business dealing with alcohol. Often, you'll see a sign on the door telling you no weapons are allowed. Alternatively, signs may be posted, saying "51% of alcohol is served here" to indicate that you cannot carry a weapon into the venue. Breaking these rules is considered a violation of the law.

Specific rules and regulations vary from state to state, so it is best to check with your local police department or search the Web for any new laws, such as the one Arizona passed to allow weapons being carried in bars. While other states are contemplating passing it as well, there are a lot of issues to be resolved, and many people are worried about possible negative outcomes. Remember, carrying a gun into a bar is risky business whether or not it is approved by law, because weapons and alcohol is often a volatile combination.

TRAVELS

If you travel to another state on vacation or a business trip, you will need to know the specific laws that apply there, even if you have a CWL in your home state.

When flying on an airplane with a gun, the weapon must be checked in as baggage—unloaded, with the ammunition in a separate bag, not in the same case. It is vital to have the weapon, such as a rifle or shotgun, in a locked case; if it is a pistol, it should be in a soft case with a lock to prevent any tampering. Declare your weapon at the airline counter and make certain to get a claim form receipt acknowledging that you are carrying a weapon. Most airlines have their own set of rules. In order to play it safe, check with your particular carrier or go online to find out the specific terms and conditions for checking in a weapon.

POLICE ENCOUNTERS

Imagine you get pulled over for speeding. The officer asks for your license and registration. You have a weapon sitting on the seat next to you or in the glove compartment, and you aren't sure whether to mention it or not. Below are the procedures to follow.

As soon as the officer approaches your window, tell him or her that you have a CWL and you have the weapon with you (loaded or unloaded). Be sure to keep your hands visible, prefer-ably on the steering wheel, and follow the officer's instructions. For instance, he may ask you to unload the gun immediately. You are required by law to follow his requests. More than likely, the officer will simply ask you not to touch your weapon. He will ask you for your CWL—you are required to carry it with you at all times—to ascertain that you're authorized to carry a weapon.

WEAPON TYPES

In most cases when you take a regular concealed handgun course, your permit allows you to carry a revolver or a semi-auto-matic. You must pass a proficiency test for whichever weapon you'll be using. Revolvers allow you to simply point and shoot. With a semi-automatic, you first need to cock it back to make sure there's a bullet in the chamber. This can be tricky, and if the weapon does not have a safety mechanism, it could accidentally discharge. Carrying a weapon with a bullet situated in the chamber is recommended be-cause to shoot, all you have to do is take the safety off and squeeze the trigger. The other rounds will automatically re-chamber until there are no more bullets left in the weapon.

I strongly suggest you take a course on semi-automatic weap-on instruction and care. After discharging your weapon you must take it apart and clean out any gun powder residue to keep it in good functioning order and prevent any misfiring in the future. There are gun-cleaning kits and lubricants for sale at most sporting goods stores. A well-functioning weapon could be the difference between life and death, as all police officers know. As a licensed carrier, the same holds true for you as well.

LIABILITIES

Disobeying the rules associated with carrying a weapon can be harmful or even deadly to you and others. You need to know when to draw and when not to. Often people will tell you they have a gun when they really don't. Until you see their weapon or they are actually causing bodily harm to others, you cannot legally draw your own gun and shoot them. If you do, you may end up in court, or worse…in prison.

When a problem arises, you want to be as calm as possible. Attempt to handle the situation without the use of deadly force. Follow the guidelines you were taught and make the correct decisions based on your training. Think about whether using your weapon will put other innocent people at risk and weigh all circumstances before going into action.

If you've been drinking alcohol, you need to leave your weapon holstered. Even if you feel you are in complete control and have only had a beer or two, under the law, you cannot use your weapon. If you need help in such circumstances, call the police and let them handle the situation.

WEAPONS ON DISPLAY

If you're wondering if you can display your weapon on your body, the answer is no. The permit says "concealed" for a reason. Remember, you're not a police officer. You are a citizen given the right to carry a concealed weapon to protect yourself and others around you. Showing it off is against the law.

Always keep your weapon where it's not in danger of being used by someone else. If someone starts playing with it and gets hurt, you could have criminal and civil charges brought against you. Do NOT let your friends carry your weapon. They did not pass the test and did not qualify to handle the weapon as you did.

EXTRA INSURANCE

It's probably a good idea to take out extra insurance when you carry a gun in the event that something happens and someone gets hurt due to your negligence. It's vital to remember that when you carry a weapon it's your responsibility to keep it away from others. However, accidents can happen easily and quickly.

In 2008, Plaxico Burress, a New York Giants football star accidently shot himself in the right thigh when he brought his Glock pistol illegally into a Manhattan nightclub (he had an expired CWL from Florida, but no New York license). He had the gun tucked into the waistband of his sweatpants. When it began to slide down his leg, he apparently reached for it, and it went off. The injury was not serious, and he was released from the hospital the next day. Soon after, he was indicted for illegal possession of a weapon and reckless endangerment, both felonies, and served two years in prison until his release in June of 2011.

In that case, Burress only hurt himself, but when others are involved, things can get more serious.

Imagine you arrive at your house after work. You notice the quiet atmosphere when the phone starts to ring in the kitchen. Thinking your wife and kids haven't come home yet, you lay your gun on the coffee table and go to answer the phone. In the meantime, your children run into the house with a neighborhood friend. While your children understand they are prohibited to touch your weapon, the other child doesn't know that. He picks up the gun too quickly and accidentally shoots himself in the foot. You are responsible because you left the weapon where a young child could reach it and get hurt. Thus, you may need extra insurance to protect yourself in case the child's parents sue.

GETTING INVOLVED

If a gunfight occurs when you are present and you feel comfortable intervening, this is where your training can become useful.

You have the responsibility to step in and use your weapon to protect the victim before the authorities arrive. But make no mistake. Even if things go smoothly, you may be more upset than you know.

Police officers are often required to go through psychological counseling after experiencing a situation in which a gunfight occurred and someone was shot. If something like that happens in your life, give yourself a few weeks to allow your emotions to settle before carrying your weapon again.

PRACTICE

It's your duty to make sure your gun functions properly at all times. You must go to the shooting range to keep your skills up to par. As I said earlier, I cannot impress upon you enough how critical it is to practice. You want to get to the point where drawing and shooting become as easy and natural as tying your shoelaces. If you are going to carry a gun, only the best training and practice will prepare you for that time when you have to go into action. At that point, you will have only seconds to weigh your options and decide if the police better handle the situation or if you should intervene. And if you decide to go ahead, you don't want to have to think about how to draw and operate your gun.

CONCLUSION

If you dislike the idea of having a concealed weapon, there are other options for you to consider, as discussed earlier in the chapter. After all, if you're uncomfortable with carrying and using a gun, there is no reason you should. Guns are serious weapons and should only be handled by those who feel confident they can do so in a safe manner.

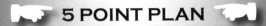

5 POINT PLAN

1. Consider taking a self-defense course, both for the skills and for the benefits of toughening up your mental attitude.

2. Tasers, mace and pepper spray can all be helpful for personal defense, but only if you've practiced using them.

3. If you decide to go for a concealed weapon license, realize that unless you can handle a gun well, it may become a liability.

4. Consider taking out extra insurance in case someone gets hurt from your weapon accidentally.

5. Practice drawing your weapon frequently and go to a shooting range at least two to three times a month.

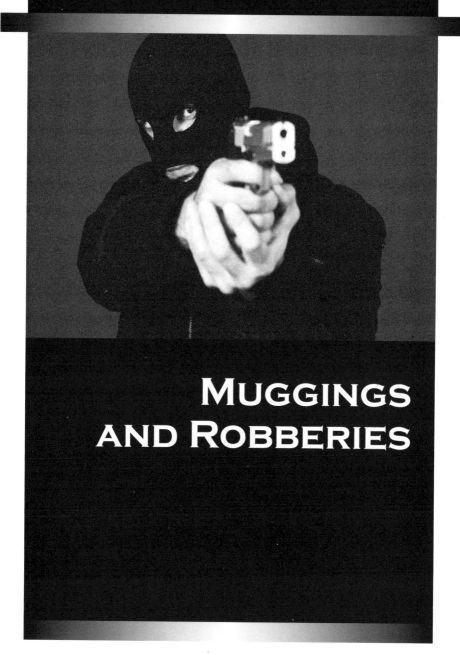

Chapter 9

MUGGINGS AND ROBBERIES

According to FBI crime statistics, more than 10 million people in the United States are victims of crime every year. That represents about 3% of the population. Of those, nearly 1.3 million are victims of violent crime.

The trauma of the event and the aftermath can be difficult to deal with. Depending on what happened, you may start to question your assumptions about yourself and the world you live in. You may not fully understand your responses both during the crime and afterwards. Even if you haven't been physically hurt, feelings of helplessness, fear, guilt, anger and rage may surprise you and, at times, threaten to overwhelm you. Add to that the difficulties of talking to the police, dealing with legal and insurance matters, and facing the personal problems that can come with being a crime victim; it is a very stressful time at best.

Take the case of a young woman who was mugged in her apartment building in New York City. There was no security guard at the downstairs entrance door, and when she got on the elevator, a young man quickly came in after her, held a knife to her throat and demanded her purse. She complied, and the assailant got off on the next floor. She was unharmed, but shaken. It all happened so fast that the only thing she remembered was the sneakers of her assailant. What she didn't count on was that for months, whenever she saw a man wearing sneakers, she experienced a jolt of fear and anxiety. After talking about it with friends and a counselor, that reaction gradually disappeared, and she started to feel in control of her life again.

DON'T BLAME YOURSELF

Under no circumstances should you reprimand yourself for what happened to you. If, after reading some of the chapters in this book, you are telling yourself, "I should have done this or that," stop and rephrase. Make it, "Up to now, I have done this. From now on,

I would want to do this or that." There is no way you could have acted based on information you did not have at the time, and so you shouldn't blame yourself.

Similarly, under no circumstances should you acquiesce to others trying to make you feel guilty or responsible for the crime. You were not at fault! You did nothing wrong! No crime can ever be justified by blaming the victim.

Here is another way to look at the situation. There are essentially three issues to consider if you become the victim of a crime:

- What to do when it happens.

- What to do immediately after the crime has occurred.

- How to cope with the long-term aftermath.

Let's review each of them in order.

WHEN IT HAPPENS

Robberies happen every day across the country. Certain people are more likely to experience robberies—those who work in retail and service industries, at convenient stores or at banks. However, even a woman walking down the street can get mugged and have her purse snatched any day of the week. Depending on the situation, there are different ways to respond.

If you're in a crowded place, the best response is to make a lot of noise. If you scream, shout or act crazy, it will attract the attention of others and may be enough to scare the culprit away. If you are being attacked and think you can put distance between yourself and your assailant, fight back. If you are able to call for help, don't yell "rape!" Yell "fire!" People will come more quickly to your assistance and may help you foil your attacker.

But if you're alone in an isolated area, it is usually better to give up the purse rather than fight for it. Be aware that the most common response when someone tries to take something that belongs to you is to resist. But doing so may put you in greater danger. The best course of action is to hand over the item the robber is demanding and get away as quickly as possible. Similarly, if someone pulls a knife or gun on you, the best course of action is not to offer any resistance.

As an overall preparation, I would suggest having emergency response numbers on speed dial on your cell phone, so you can press the button at the earliest sign of trouble. If nothing else, the crime will be recorded by the police on a 911 call. They may be able to use that recording later on to catch the bad guys using voice recognition devices or because the attackers had unusual accents.

As the crime is taking place, focus on what is actually happening around you. Even though you'll be nervous, try to memorize any details about your assailant—from physical features, like height, weight, eye color, facial hair, scars or tattoos, to clothes and behavior, including jewelry and distinctive accents. Anything you can remember will give the police a head start on catching the criminal. Anything you can do to assist in getting these people off the street will be good for the entire community.

If you get held up at work, don't try to become a hero. Most companies make it a policy, in case of a robbery, for their employees to hand over all the money. It's the safest course of action. If an employee resists, the robber, who may be already on edge, might get angry and hurt someone. Money can be replaced, and most businesses are insured against robberies. Just as in a street crime, if you find yourself caught in such a situation, try to remember any special features of the robbers to report to the police when they come to investigate.

IMMEDIATELY AFTER THE CRIME

While most robbers will take what they want and run away, you should not linger at the crime scene, in case they decide to hang around for further mischief and turn you into a more serious crime victim. Then, as soon as you can, find a police officer or call 911 to report the crime.

In a calm voice, report your location and give a detailed description of the criminals. Speak clearly and slowly. If you have to repeat yourself, you'll be giving the criminals more time to escape. In most areas, 911 dispatchers will be able to find your location instantly, whether you tell it to them or not. They are tied into GPS, which will tell them your exact location if you're using your cell phone or are calling from a pay phone. So, don't be worried if you don't know where you are during the call.

If you are a female and have been assaulted or raped, request a female officer to talk to. It is your right to choose who you want to do your investigation and you need to have someone with whom you can feel comfortable.

If you have been victimized in any other way—whether in a drive-by shooting or a home invasion—first make sure you are no longer under attack. Usually, things happen quickly and are over before you know it. Check to see if you or family members have been physically hurt. If that is the case, try to get immediate help from others nearby and then call 911 for an ambulance and the police.

If you or members of your family aren't hurt, make sure there isn't someone still in the house waiting to get away. After going through the place room by room, start to estimate the damage.

Start making calls to repair any property damage from a security standpoint. If there was a home invasion, call a locksmith immediately to replace the locks and fix the door so that you can have some form of protection for the rest of the night. Even if the crime occurred during the day, make sure to get the property secured right away. You never know if someone else might be waiting for the right moment to loot your home and cause further harm to you or your family.

The most important thing is that you and any other family members or friends involved are OK. Be aware that you or a member of your family may go into shock in response to what happened. They may complain of being cold and nauseous, and begin to shake. Get blankets to keep them warm. You can also trust that the authorities and EMT personnel have the training and expertise to take care of them in the best possible way.

As soon as you're done talking to the police, contact your bank and credit card companies to cancel all debit and credit cards. Keep photocopies of all your credit cards at your house, in a safe location. That way, if someone snatches your wallet, you can quickly access all information and know exactly what cards to call about.

Do not touch anything or try to clean up—that may destroy valuable evidence. Take pictures of anything you can right away, because when the police get there they will ask you to vacate the premises until they have determined whether or not there is any evidence that can lead to the conviction of the criminals when they are caught.

While that is going on, search your schedule and movements for clues of any suspicious or erratic behavior that you may have noticed prior to the attack. Retrace your steps and identify anything odd that might suggest the attack was planned, not random, and let the police know right away.

COPING WITH THE LONG-TERM AFTERMATH

Surviving the crime is just the first step on the road to recovery. But what happens afterward? Being a victim can haunt you for a long time and in unexpected ways. You may experience angry fantasies of wanting to maim or kill your assailants. Feelings of guilt, depression, helplessness and worthlessness are not uncommon.

If you have been the victim of a home invasion, for example, you're going to feel vulnerable and unsafe for a long period of time.

You may suffer from "Why Me?" Syndrome, feel sorry for yourself and fall into the stereotypical victim mindset. Feeling defenseless, you may let your guard down, making you an easy target for a second attack. You may live in fear and feel violated for some time.

There is nothing wrong with such reactions—they are normal—but it is important not to stay stuck with them for too long. The goal should be to make sure that you are more prepared if this were to happen to you again. When you walk away from a bad experience that could have cost you your life, you need to treat it as a gift that provides you the opportunity for a second chance. You owe it to yourself to become prepared and to prepare others.

How can you do this?

Many cities now offer victim assistance programs, generally consisting of groups in which previously victimized people attempt to help each other. Many organizations offer counseling services for victims of trauma and abuse. Depending on your religion, talking to a priest, minister or rabbi can also be helpful. Above all, don't feel you have to suffer in silence or overcome your trauma all by yourself.

At the same time, regardless of how you feel, it is helpful to take measures to protect yourself in the future, even if you have to force yourself to do so for a while. Until you can feel safe in your home, for example, the sense of having been violated isn't likely to go away.

The good news is that you can protect yourself and start to feel safe quickly after a home invasion. We have already talked about purchasing solid doors and high-security locks, creating a safe room in the house, and stocking it with appropriate tools for safety and defense, including cell phones, flashlights and, if you so choose, weapons. You can also install a security system on all windows and check to be sure your outdoor areas are well-lit and secure. You also might want to look into getting a stronger gate for your fence with a larger lock. In addition, you can get motion sensitive lighting so it looks like your house is dark until the mechanism registers movement, and the lights pop on. Research what items will protect you, your family and your property best. Knowing that no one can enter your home without you being well aware of it can help you feel secure and get a solid night's sleep again.

Inform your neighbors of what happened and let them help you if they offer assistance in the future. Don't go out alone. Always have at least one other person with you for a while. If you live alone, consider getting a roommate.

If you have been robbed or assaulted, contact the police department about taking a self-defense class. If you live in a neighborhood with a high crime rate and limited options in the matter of security, you may want to consider applying for a concealed weapon permit and get proper training in the use of a gun. These precautions will protect you and give you the peace of mind you need. When you begin to feel that you can handle bad situations, your fear will disappear.

CONCLUSION

The best way to help yourself is to become more in control. If you have been going through the day on autopilot with minimal awareness of your surroundings, make a point of paying more attention. The manner in which you handle yourself can either put you in a weak position, inviting criminals to make you their prey for another attack, or signal to them that you're not a good candidate for them to victimize. Show them that you are strong and ready to take care of yourself.

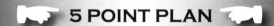

5 POINT PLAN

1. Under no circumstances should you blame yourself for being the victim of a crime.

2. If attacked for any reason, shout and yell "fire!" if you're in a crowd. If alone, do what the attacker says.

3. Afterward, call 911 as soon as you can to report the crime.

4. Report credit cards and other documents stolen right away.

5. Be aware that you may have negative, even debilitating, reactions to what happened for a long time, and consider getting counseling to restore your balance and move forward in a positive manner.

Chapter 10

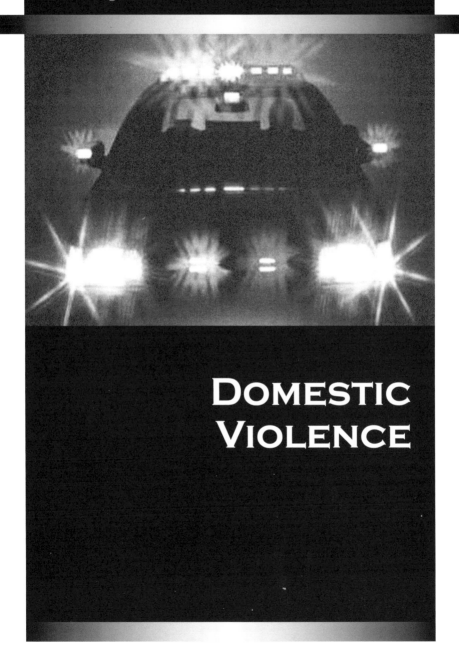

DOMESTIC VIOLENCE

Domestic violence can be like a snake in the grass, lying hidden and dormant for some time, and then biting you when you're least expecting it. Sometimes good relationships turn bad when a family member loses his or her job and turns to drugs or alcohol to numb the anxiety, pain and despair. The problem is that such "fixes" can provide some emotional relief, but they can also trigger violent behavior.

In many cases, family violence is endemic, however, and the abuse goes on for a number of years, often ending in crippling injuries or even death.

Sometimes, after a difficult breakup, the person who was left becomes angry and vengeful, stalking, assaulting and even killing his former spouse. We have all heard or read about cases in which someone took out a restraining order after repeated attacks, but to no avail because the perpetrator simply ignored it and came back to cause further harm and even death.

The prevalence of domestic violence in the United States is overwhelming. If it were classified as a disease, we would call it an epidemic and work overtime to find an antidote, but because domestic abuse takes place in the privacy of people's homes, it remains out of sight and concealed from public scrutiny and outrage.

Both men and women can be victims of domestic abuse, but let's be clear: Most of the violence is directed against women. Nearly one in four women—that is 25%—reports having been raped and/or physically assaulted by a current or former spouse, partner, boyfriend or acquaintance at some point in life. For men, the figure is 7.6%. Indeed, women represent 84% of all spouse abuse victims.

While there has been some progress in calling attention to the problem during the past decades—setting up hotlines and creating shelters for victims of domestic abuse, for example—the figures continue to be daunting:

- On average in the United States, more than three women a day are murdered by their husbands or boyfriends.

- Women experience two million injuries from intimate partner violence each year.

- In 2007, there were more than 500 rapes/sexual assaults per day.

- More than 50% of the men who assaulted their wives also beat their children.

- Annually, between 3.3 and 10 million children witness abuse at home.

- While women of all ages are at risk for domestic violence, 20- to 24-year-olds are most affected. These women, as a group, also experience the highest rates of rape and sexual assault.

- There are serious health issues related to physical abuse. Women who have suffered domestic violence are 80% more likely to have a stroke, 70% more likely to have heart disease, and 60% more likely to have asthma than women who have not experienced domestic violence.

DON'T ACCEPT VERBAL ABUSE

Physical violence is not the only type of abuse. Verbal abuse is also common and its effect is harmful, too. When someone in a position of authority, such as a parent or spouse, continually acts in an insulting manner and uses words to belittle and dress others down, in time the victims will accept that negative point of view and treatment as the truth. They may come to feel that they are useless and life is worthless. They may believe that their spouse or parent doesn't love them, and that it is their fault. In the end they may turn to drugs and alcohol for relief. Children may join gangs or socialize with criminal friends who will lead them down the wrong path.

Children treated disrespectfully can quickly become disrespectful themselves and will no longer listen to their parents or other authorities. Verbally abusing a child creates another member of society who will continue the cycle of violence and who is likely to use the same approach with his children. It is surely not an accident that 100% of the criminals on death row suffered significant physical and emotional abuse as children; and while such abuse doesn't lead everyone to become a criminal or murderer, it is certainly not a positive factor for anyone.

CHILDREN IN VIOLENT HOUSEHOLDS

When children are in the presence of family violence, it can leave deep emotional scars. They are involved even if the parents try to keep it a secret—children know what's happening even if they can't understand what it means. Therefore, it is important to acknowledge that there is a problem. Make sure your children understand that it is not their fault. Young children, especially, personalize things and think they are responsible for everything in their surroundings. Addressing the problem by sharing your plans to fix it is essential, too, in order to keep your children safe from the emotional effects of violence.

CHILDREN AS VICTIMS OF DOMESTIC VIOLENCE

Sometimes the abusing adult feels the best way to take advantage of his spouse is to harm the kids. This is when things really get ugly and hurtful, because children are vulnerable and unable to protect themselves. I have come upon situations in which a child was literally thrown against a wall or beaten to the point where she required admission to the hospital.

Doctors and nurses are required by law to report violence against children, so in such circumstances the perpetrator is likely to have to deal with the authorities. If the abuse keeps happening, the children may be taken away and placed with foster parents. Often, they will leave home willingly because they don't feel any protection or safety there. Once again, they may feel there is no one there who loves them.

Can children ever feel safe again after experiencing physical and mental abuse? Yes, but it will take time. They will start to feel secure again only if there's some consistency in their lives. They should be told that the things that happened to them were wrong. When they realize someone is concerned about their well-being and safety and that abuse will no longer be tolerated, they can start the process of slowly trusting others again and believing that they are OK.

COPING WITH DOMESTIC VIOLENCE

Domestic abuse is not so different from a home invasion that has turned violent, except that the criminal is an intimate family member. If you are one of the millions who suffer from domestic abuse and happen to read this chapter, make a decision to become active in your own defense. For many, that is the first and most critical step. If you feel threatened in your home by another family member or worry about your children being abused, don't wait and hope that it magically will go away. Start taking proactive measures to defend yourself.

The most important thing you can do is remove yourself and your children from the scene to a place of safety. Consider where you could turn if you needed to flee quickly to take refuge. It could be a safe room in your home, or it could be a neighbor's house.

If you feel you are at risk of domestic abuse, you need to be aware of the dangers of staying in the home and become prepared for possible violence in the future. You may want to leave and go to a shelter. There you will be safe in the short run and can get help with counseling and legal issues as well. Above all, you will experience relief when you no longer feel alone and carry the burden all by yourself.

If you decide to stay in your home, you may need to hire an attorney who will help you get a restraining order to keep the criminal away from you and your property. Be aware, though, that such an order provides only limited protection. Chances are, someone who assaulted you will try to cause you bodily harm again or at least try to destroy your property. If he shows up, will you have enough time to call the police? If he arrives with a gun, how will you defend yourself?

For ultimate safety, you'll want to have a barrier between you and the perpetrator. Involve your neighbors; inform them of what has happened and when, and let them help you in the future. If you have a restraining order, alert them to that fact and ask them to warn you and call 911 if they see the assailant in the neighborhood.

Most importantly, protect yourself by creating a safe room in the house with a high-security locking device that can withstand a kick from a man who is boiling over with rage and anger.

Let's take a typical scenario—one in which life and death are not at stake, but which may result in a great deal of physical harm for you.

Imagine your partner has been out drinking and comes home staggering and irritated. It looks like he may lose his temper if he notices you just breathing in his direction. The most important thing to remember in such situations is that you cannot reason with anyone under the influence of drugs and alcohol when they're at the point of exploding. Even if you retreat to another room in the home to get away, things can get worse: The attacker may get furious and kick in the door to get to you.

In the past, you probably felt that there was no alterative and nowhere to go. If you have set up a safe room with a high-security lock that can withstand up to 4,000 pounds of force, however, you can retreat there and give your angry spouse time to cool off and get back to his senses. Make sure, though, that the door to the room is solid core, not hollow like most interior doors. Being able to retreat to a safe room with your children is the best way to keep yourself protected against harm. While going to a neighbor's house is also a good idea, there is the danger that your violent partner will grab you on your way out the door. It's much easier to get to a "safe room" inside the house and call for help from there.

You might also want to install a high-security lock on the front door designed to prevent home invasions. If you engage its "lock out" feature, the perpetrator cannot get into your home even with his own key! Chances are he will go to the car and sleep it off. If he attempts to get in another way—through a window, for example—you will have enough time to retreat to your safe room, call the police and have him arrested. In fact, when someone is locked out in this manner and tries to get in by force, he is technically guilty of criminal trespassing. If he calls the police and claims that he cannot get in to his own house, he will only dig himself into deeper trouble. When the officers arrive on the scene and discover that the caller is drunk, they will arrest him and charge him with public intoxication in most cases.

Often, when the person sobers up and realizes he was acting wrongly, he may say something like, "Please forgive my bad behavior," and expect you to give in. But make no mistake. You need help in the long run. Don't assume the problem will go away. You may feel that you can't let anyone else know about your personal problems, but there are other people who can relate to your crisis and offer sound advice. Don't allow things to get out of hand. With domestic violence, counseling is very important for everyone in the family.

CONCLUSION

I personally recommend that you allow someone with a tendency toward physical violence to remain in the house only if he demonstrates that he can control his behavior. And I suggest you inform him that if he ever becomes violent again, it's over. You will leave or have him arrested. If it happens, make good on your promise.

But I am well aware that few people are capable of such determination and follow through. It rarely happens without outside support.

The bottom line: Get help. Don't wait until it's too late.

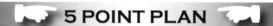

5 POINT PLAN

1. Be aware that domestic abuse can be both physical and verbal and will affect every member of the household—including children—in one way or another.

2. Domestic violence is like a home invasion, except that the criminal is a close family member.

3. As with home invasions, having solid doors and high-quality locks on the entrances to the house and a safe room inside are the first lines of defense and protection.

4. Getting a restraining order can be helpful, but will not offer protection against a determined abuser.

5. Getting counseling is critical to help break the cycle of abuse and violence.

Chapter 11

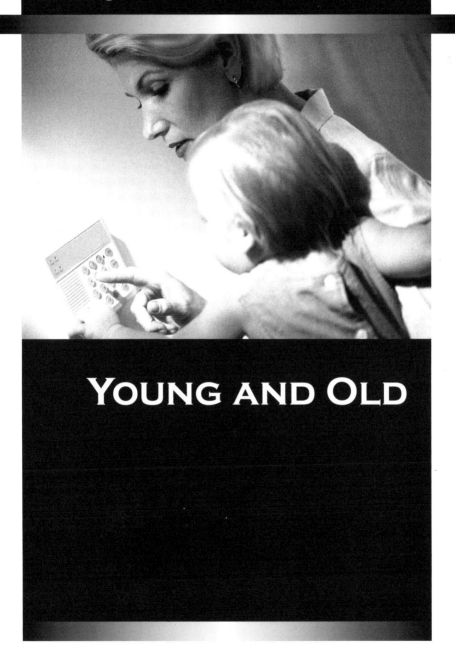

YOUNG AND OLD

When it comes to safety, youths and the elderly are two unique population groups that have distinct issues and special needs. While teens and young adults suffer the highest violent crime rates, including murder, rape and sexual assault, older citizens tend to be more the target of property crimes such as purse snatching, car theft and robbery, as well as fraud and scams.

YOUTH AND YOUNG ADULTS

When I was growing up, my parents never locked the front or back doors to the house. We played outside unsupervised for hours on end, roaming through the neighborhood and returning home only when it got dark and it was time for dinner. While there are still some parts of the United States where one can live in such an idyllic, innocent world, nowadays most cities and suburbs are more dangerous. Few parents would let their young children play alone in the yard or the street even in a quiet neighborhood or suburban subdivision. They would certainly keep an eye on them from inside the house. In many communities, the parents of grade school children take turns watching over the bus stop in the morning and afternoon when their children go to and return from school.

And for good reason. The statistics on youth crime are staggering. All parents concerned about the safety and well-being of their children should be aware of them. After all, it's the parents' job to keep their children safe and secure at all times.

Here are just a few of the startling statistics:

■ Teenagers belong to the age group that experiences the most violent crime.

■ 16- to 19-year-old girls represent the second largest group of rape and sexual assault victims.

■ Youngsters are the largest group being stalked.

■ The growing incidents of cyber crimes, such as stalking via chat rooms and Facebook, as well as cyberbullying, affect teens more than any other age group.

PROTECT YOUR CHILDREN

We've already discussed the importance of being aware of what is going on in your community by checking with police, reading newspapers, watching television news programs and looking at websites that list ex-cons, such as child molesters, and their addresses, so you can determine if any live close by. Be sure your young children are aware of the dangers of talking to strangers, no matter how charming or friendly they may seem.

But while close supervision and paying attention works well with young children, when they get to be teenagers and older, things become more challenging. High school and early college is a time when youngsters start the process of separating themselves from their parents by testing boundaries. Sometimes, this takes the form of rebellious behavior that can border on the obnoxious; sometimes it's just a matter of exploration, experimentation and "pushing the envelope." I have met a number of "Goth" kids who are "A" students and perfectly nice people underneath all the black lipstick, eye shadow and nail polish. Often teenagers will behave flagrantly or say outrageous things just to see what kind of reaction they'll get from adults. When that feedback is negative, they might backpedal and say they didn't mean it. And in most cases, they honestly didn't because they are still in the process of figuring out who they are, still maturing and growing, so it's not a bad idea to cut them some slack.

The difficulty is that this normal process also means teenagers are less likely to listen to adults and heed legitimate warnings. Yet, while they may seem sophisticated and can run circles around their parents when it comes to using computers and the Internet, they still have limited life experience. At a time when they want to assert their independence, they are also most vulnerable to being taken advantage of by "cool" friends and unscrupulous predators and criminals. That is why parents and mentors are so important at this stage of their development.

GANGS

If there are gangs in your area—they exist in many small towns and suburbs now, not just in big cities—they can present problems on the way to and from school and even during school hours. Parents should strongly discourage their children from getting involved in any gang activity.

BE AWARE

Children should know what to do if they become a victim of a crime, or if they are home alone and an intruder enters the house (see Chapters 4 and 6 for further details). They might enroll in a self-defense course, so they can physically protect themselves, if necessary. Most importantly, they need to know if there are particular issues in the community of which they should be aware. Sheltering children from unpleasant news is commendable, but not in the case when there's a criminal loose in a neighborhood or a child molester living nearby. At those times, it's best for parents to inform their children in an age-appropriate manner.

Your children should always be aware of their surroundings and never wander around the neighborhood alone. That goes for teenagers as well, not just younger children. There have been a number of unfortunate instances in which middle or high school girls walking down the street were assaulted and/or kidnapped in broad daylight by an older predator. Traveling in groups is much safer and can help prevent crimes involving thousands of children each year. At night, this is a must!

DATING

When it comes to dating, parents should make their children aware of potential dangers. Sexual assault and rape can occur within what may seem like "normal" teen relationships. Parents of teenage daughters should be honest about the possible risks associated with dating and how to best protect themselves. One simple tip: Never leave your drink or food alone when you go to the restroom, for example. Some teenage boys or young men will take the opportunity to lace them with "date rape" drugs in order to take advantage later on. If you have had to step away, get a new drink. This is good advice for college students and women in their 20s as well.

CYBER CRIMES

Adult predators hooking up with minors in online chat rooms has been a problem for some time, but cyberbullying is a recent phenomenon that has become a nightmare for many youngsters. Part of the difficulty is that the Internet grants a great deal of anonymity to bullies and child molesters. They can make up fake or "dummy" account names, and some websites are reluctant to reveal their real identities, citing right to privacy issues. In a recent case, a small group of troublemakers stole a student's identity, made up a fake profile for him on Facebook, and posted rude and mean-spirited remarks about other students in school. As a result, the unsuspecting student got into trouble and was shunned by his classmates. It was only because of his mother's relentless determination that the real culprits were tracked down and her son's name was cleared.

Be sure to encourage your children to let you know if they are the victim of cyberbullying. If you end up having to deal with such a situation, don't be shy. Report it to the police. You may have to go as far as hiring a detective to track down the perpetrators. Remember, they have committed a crime even if they claim it was just a prank. If it turns out that they are friends or schoolmates of your child, you may be met with denial or attempts to belittle you when confronting the parents of the culprits and demanding an apology. Also be aware that your child needs a great deal of support during this ordeal. The process can drag on for some time and you may want to hire a counselor to help with all the conflicting emotions that surface.

Fortunately, some of the social network sites are beginning to deal with this problem more directly, making it easier to remove offensive messages and cooperating with the authorities in cases of identity theft and cyber-stalking.

TEACH YOUR CHILDREN RIGHT FROM WRONG

There is another important issue that may occur as children grow older, and can throw parents for a loop: what to do when they land in hot water themselves—whether it's a speeding ticket, a car accident, a case of vandalism, or worse.

If your children get into trouble, don't react with hurt, disappointment or anger. Use it as an opportunity for them to learn about the curveballs life can throw at them. As a parent, the important things to remember are that you not only know more than your kids, but you also are older and (hopefully) wiser than them. You might try to approach the inevitably awkward conversation regarding what happened and what to do about it with understanding, a sense of humor and love. Most kids will listen to you if they sense that you are being straight with them, care for them and have their best interest at heart.

Not all issues can be resolved through conversations, however. As a parent, you should be prepared to step up as a disciplinarian, as needed. It is your job to teach youngsters the difference between right and wrong when they don't conduct themselves properly and get into trouble. But you can be firm without being verbally or physically abusive. Use the simple technique of taking away privileges when they misbehave. Take the cell phone away for a week.

Restrict them by saying they aren't allowed to be with their friends. The first time they'll be shocked, but it will have a major impact on them; it will give them a chance to think about their bad behavior and realize that there are consequences.

PURSUE PREVENTIVE MEASURES

Obviously, the best solution is to nip problems in the bud, before children get themselves into trouble. When you don't like the people your children are hanging around with, voice your concern and say, "I'm not trying to choose your friends, but I expect you to adhere to certain basic rules of right and wrong, and I won't accept less from you." Tell them they are "good" children and you don't want them to get in trouble for something a friend does. Teach them about the principle of guilt by association, even when they have done nothing wrong themselves.

Peer pressure can be a powerful tool of persuasion; unless children realize that they need to resist bad influences, it can be a difficult challenge. In my law enforcement experience, I've dealt with a large number of troubled youngsters at a juvenile youth program. Most of them were trying to find themselves as people, test their boundaries and return to the normal avenues of society. It's not always easy for them to accept responsibility for what they did and it may take considerable time before they come around.

In such cases, parents can often benefit by involving expert counselors. Few of us are prepared for extraordinary circumstances when they happen with our children for the first time, and none of us are trained what to do if it becomes a chronic problem. In extreme cases, the best course of action may be to remove the child from his normal surroundings and enroll him in a special prep school where oversight is more stringent and rules are consistently enforced, but they can be costly and require careful consideration and planning.

THE ELDERLY

Many older people and their families worry about crime, and for good reason. The elderly may be well organized as a group, through AARP, for example, and represent a powerful political bloc in our society, but as individuals they are more vulnerable than other segments of the population. Many fear for their physical safety, especially when they live alone, despite the fact that violent crimes against them are comparatively rare in relation to other age groups.

Still, the crimes that can and do happen to them pose serious concerns. An older person is more likely to be seriously hurt when involved in a physical crime than someone who is younger. And according to AARP studies, in some categories—notably fraud and scams, purse snatching, pickpocketing, theft of checks from the mail, and mistreatment in long-term care settings—the elderly lead the statistics.

When serious crimes such as robbery or home invasion do occur, the damage and loss of possessions may be worse emotionally for an older person rather than financially or physically. The victim may never feel safe in his or her living quarters again, leading to increased worry, and diminished pleasure and quality of life.

Living in fear of crime is never a good thing, whether legitimate or imaginary, and it should not stop you from enjoying life. It does make sense to be extra careful and, as I have mentioned throughout this book, aware of your surroundings. At the same time, there are many things you can do to prevent becoming a victim of crime and stay safe. A number of them have been covered before in earlier chapters, but they bear repeating as a reminder.

Always keep your entry doors and windows locked, whether you are in your home or not. High-security locks on the front and back doors will go a long way to ease your mind. Installing a good alarm system may also be beneficial for when you are not at home.

Make sure all walkways, driveways and outside doorways around your home are well-lit at night. Often, such illumination will be a strong deterrent, as criminals prefer to work unseen in the dark.

Do not open the front door to any stranger without first demanding proper identification. Scam artists and robbers have been known to pose as repairmen, meter readers for utility companies, delivery men for FedEx or UPS, and even police officers. Make sure you see their badge or ID card first. Ask for packages to be left at the door and take them inside after the deliveryman has left. If you feel at all uneasy, don't open the door!

BE STREET SMART

Be especially aware of your surroundings when you go out. Don't go out alone, especially at night. Develop a buddy system with friends and neighbors.

If you're driving, keep your car doors locked at all times, and do not roll down your window for strangers. Avoid dark streets and parking lots; park in well-lit areas instead.

If you are carrying a purse, put the strap over your shoulder and across your chest, so that it can't be snatched easily. While there are stories of 80-year-olds resisting a robber successfully—and they invariably make the nightly TV news—in general it is best to hand over your cash and whatever else the robber demands. You're less likely to suffer physical harm.

BE SAFE WITH YOUR MONEY

Do not keep large amounts of money in your house. Have monthly pension or social security checks sent to the bank for direct deposit. Keep your checkbook and credit cards in separate places. That will make it harder for a thief to forge your signature successfully.

When going to the bank, vary your routine. Go on different days and at different times each week.

Carry your wallet and credit cards on you in an inside pocket, not in your purse. Avoid having a lot of cash with you.

Do not give your credit card or bank account number to anyone who calls you on the telephone, even if they claim they are from your bank. Similarly, do not respond to e-mails asking for any of your financial information. These are attempts by scam artists to take advantage of you. Just hang up on telephone salespeople. Nothing you need is sold exclusively over the phone. You can always purchase it in person or from a reputable Internet website.

Be on the alert for scam artists in person, via the telephone or on the Internet, promising you money or great investment opportunities. If a deal sounds too good to be true, it probably is. That's how Arthur Nadel and Bernard Madoff "made off" with investors' funds—by promising astronomical returns on their money. And look what it got them.

DON'T TOLERATE ELDER ABUSE

It is a terrible reflection on humanity, but there are people who mistreat the elderly in their care, often at a time when they are most helpless and unable to do anything about it. Elder abuse can take many forms and can happen anywhere. Physical harm, sexual assault, neglect and theft of money and valuables can occur as easily at home, involving family members and friends, as in a nursing home by supposedly professional caregivers.

Whatever the case may be, it is a crime, and reporting such abuse is not only a moral obligation, but in most states, a legal responsibility as well. Whether it has happened to you yourself or someone else, it is important to report it to the police right away. You can also contact your local or state Adult Protective Services program for help.

If you've been physically harmed, see your doctor as soon as possible. In some situations, you may need to hire an attorney to take legal action.

As a Family Member

With Baby Boomers increasingly having to take care of their aging parents, there are some basic routines and procedures that can help ensure their safety.

Besides making sure that a senior's residence is safe, it's important for family members to do routine monitoring. Set up "check in" times when a senior agrees to be home for a phone call or personal visit from a family member. You may want to do this several times a day.

If you can afford it, consider hiring a part-time or full-time adult sitter or caretaker to come in during the day to help the senior maintain safety. In some cases, round the clock, seven days a week service may be required.

There are also monitoring services such as Life Alert that allow the senior to contact help at the push of a button. It requires wearing a bracelet or necklace that can be used to call for help if there is a fire, a medical emergency or a home invasion.

One area in which elder safety can be compromised is while driving. Many seniors don't want to give up the freedom that having a car represents. However, it is critical that family members monitor the driving abilities of their elderly parents. If they are unable to drive safely or are getting lost en route to various places, you may have to ask them to give up their license. This can be a difficult conversation and cause considerable stress when trying to figure out how to cope with the loss of a car. Many towns have excellent public transportation systems, which can give senior citizens the freedom they desire without putting them and others on the road at risk.

CONCLUSION

Since people live longer these days—those who are 100 and older are the fastest-growing age group in the United States—the issue of security for our elderly population should be one of our main concerns. Many seniors are vigorous and active well into their 90s, but only if we and they can feel confident that they are safe and taken care of is it possible for them to live their life to the fullest. Someday, we will be in their shoes. In the meantime, we should do nothing less for them than we would want for ourselves when we reach their age.

5 POINT PLAN

1. Make sure your children are aware of the potential dangers in their school and neighborhood.

2. Teach your children right from wrong.

3. The homes of seniors should be secured the way you would protect yourself from a home invasion, with alarm systems and high-quality locks.

4. Be smart with your money and look out for Internet and telephone scams.

5. For seniors living alone, their safety and health should be monitored with agreed upon "check in" phone calls or personal visits at least once a day.

Chapter 12

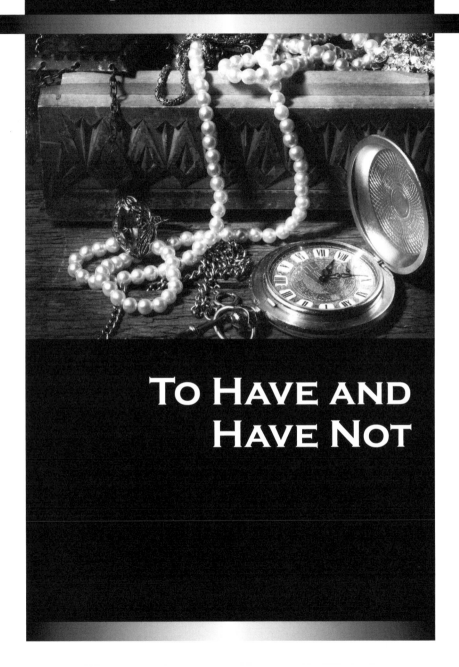

TO HAVE AND HAVE NOT

As I am writing this book, America is going through a deep recession; some economists even call it a depression. Although there are signs of a gradual recovery in some sectors of our society, the prognosis is that it will take a long time for our nation to dig itself out of the hole into which it has fallen. Hard economic times have a strong effect on public and private safety as crimes against property rise. With a growing number of people laid off from work, depleting their savings and retirement accounts, and unable to pay their bills, some of them turn to crime to make ends meet.

This is not a new phenomenon. In 17th-century England, when the economy was depressed for many years, people turned to theft and robbery even though they were capital crimes, punishable by death. Those caught and convicted were hanged and had their intestines cut out while they were still alive to display to the crowds who came to watch the executions. We consider such harsh punishment barbaric, but the point I want to make is that it did not deter others from continuing to become highwaymen and thieves, robbing travelers on the roads and burglarizing homes and estates. When the alternative is poverty and starvation, many turn to crime regardless of the consequences.

TARGETING THE WELL-OFF

A couple of years ago, the officers from my police department were called to a neighborhood in a wealthy part of town because the owner of a villa thought his house alarm had been tripped by an intruder. It turned out to be a false alarm. Over the next couple of weeks, this happened several times, and the officers dutifully returned to the home to check things out. Each time it was another false alarm. As a result, they became less vigilant. The last time it happened, they did a cursory perimeter check and knocked on the front door. When no one answered, they assumed all was well.

A few days later, during their routine rounds of the neighborhood, they noticed that newspapers were piling up on the front porch of the residence—no one had picked them up. When the officers conducted a more thorough investigation, they found that the back door had been kicked in. The homeowners, a middle-aged couple, were alive in a safe room, but terrified. They managed to escape the intruders, but not before they had been tortured and were forced to reveal their bank account numbers and the location of the key to their safe-deposit box. When the police checked further, it turned out that the box and all of their bank accounts had been cleaned out.

The criminals had done their homework. They obviously knew the comings and goings of this couple, had researched their assets, and lulled the police into paying less attention than usual. The culprits were never caught.

In our society, having class means possessing a sense of elegance and dignity; in the world of crime, "class" represents nothing more than a difference in socio-economic levels. No matter which economic class we are in, we're all affected by crime. Most violent crimes still occur between people who know each other. No matter if you are in an upper, middle or lower income level, you can be victimized. But if you're well-off, you are a bigger target and have more to lose. There are steps you can take to protect yourself.

How big a target are you?

When it comes to home invasions and other forms of robbery and theft, there are many things criminals look for when choosing their next victim. But you can be sure that they are attracted to houses that appear to hold things of value. For some criminals, the desire to have the finer things they can't afford is all the motivation they need. They see what others have and they want it for themselves. If you have a beautiful, large home, drive expensive cars and wear fancy jewelry, they could target you. If you brag about having nice electronics, including home theaters, you could make yourself susceptible to attack.

KEEP A LOW PROFILE

How noticeable are you? Do you stand out in a crowd? Do you make it obvious that you have a lot of money? It's great to work hard and reap the rewards. In fact, it may have taken you years to attain your current social and economic status, but openly displaying your wealth is like wearing a bull's-eye. If you want to be safe, it is far better not to draw attention to yourself.

Thus, it is not a good idea to mention the expensive antiques or the original oil paintings you have in your home. Keep all information on valuables and their worth to yourself or within your immediate family and friends. You never know who is listening and taking notes.

When you go out to dinner and pay with cash, don't pull out a wad of one hundred dollar bills! By showing the world you have a pocket full of money, you're inviting trouble. In today's "debit card world" people rarely carry large sums of money, and if you flash cash around, you'll be sending out invitations to every criminal in the area to take a special interest in you. Remember, your money is a private matter and is no one else's business.

If you drive an expensive car and wear extravagant clothes when you go out, people will take a closer look at you. Career criminals have a great deal of experience in detecting whether someone is a worthy target or not. They analyze the way you dress, how you act, the car you drive and where you live. They look at the friends you keep and evaluate their status as well.

Some wealthy people have personalized license plates, for example. If you are one of them, be aware that they make your car easier to identify. Criminals may use the opportunity to track you and learn your daily and weekly routine.

PROTECT YOUR HOME

Short of hiring bodyguards and security officers to protect your home around the clock, you're in the same boat as everyone else. The security alarm system you install may be state of the art, but it will function only if it is turned on. Certainly, motion detection devices around your property and highly visible security cameras at the gate and at your house can help to act as deterrents. I strongly recommend building a special safe room that can't be penetrated. Some new mansions have a concrete safe room built as part of the structure that will withstand hurricane force winds. Like the black boxes in airplanes, they are designed to survive any and all disasters.

Short of that, make sure your doors and windows are well-protected. Invest in bulletproof windows on the ground floor, and, of course, high-quality locks on all entrance doors.

CONCLUSION

Just because you can afford the better things in life, you shouldn't have to constantly look over your shoulder. But remember, wearing expensive designer clothes and 10 pounds worth of jewelry on a regular basis is similar to having a large flashing neon sign on your back that reads, "I'm loaded. Come and get me." It's better to limit displaying your possessions in public to specific events and enjoy them in the safe and secure comfort of your home.

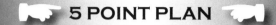

5 POINT PLAN

1. Take an inventory of yourself and your behavior to determine how much information about your possessions becomes public knowledge.

2. Avoid flashing cash or expensive items in public.

3. Consider leaving the expensive clothes and jewelry at home when you go out, unless it's for a special occasion.

4. Keep a low profile in public whenever you can.

5. Fortify your home with alarm systems, bulletproof windows and high-quality locks.

Chapter 13

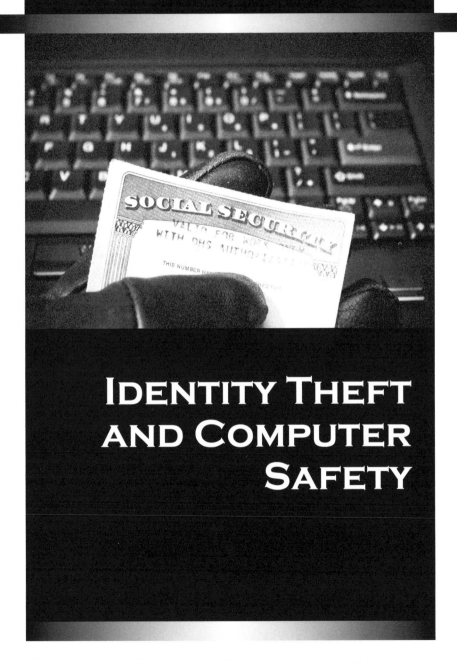

IDENTITY THEFT
AND COMPUTER
SAFETY

Over the past two decades, the Internet has exploded, and it continues to grow by leaps and bounds. From connecting families over long distances, to e-commerce, online education, new forms of entertainment and much, much more, it has become an essential part of our lives, creating wonderful opportunities for everyone. But there is a dark side, too, heightened by the relative anonymity criminals enjoy when they operate in virtual reality. Viruses and worms can crash one's computer and shut down whole websites, and child pornography, online bullying and other ugly developments keep pace with the benefits new technology has provided.

One of the most prevalent aspects has been the increase in identity theft. In less than five minutes, criminals can take your identity. They can then not only use it locally, but sell it for use anywhere in the world.

Over the course of 12 months in 2007, the Federal Trade Commission's complaint database received more than 800,000 consumer fraud and identity theft complaints. Financial losses exceeded $1.2 billion, and the problem is getting bigger all the time.

Identity theft can affect anyone at any time, and sometimes when you least expect it.

Two years ago, my wife and I went to the movies and left her laptop computer in the car. It was in a carrying case. When we got back, we saw that the car had been broken into, and the computer was gone. We never found out who stole it and didn't get it back. My wife lost a great deal of valuable data, and because she had not password protected her files, we worried that her identity was compromised. Getting another computer and recovering her documents from memory proved to be a great deal of trouble, not to mention worrying that her personal information had gotten into the wrong hands and would cause us further difficulties at some future time. Fortunately, the thief must have only been interested in what money he could get for the piece of equipment, because we have seen no fallout. We did learn our lesson, though, and have taken all the necessary safety precautions (see below).

The result can cost you money, ruin your credit and even destroy your personal reputation. When your identity is in the hands of criminals, it can be used in illegal activities such as smuggling, fraud, theft by check or the purchase of property you will be responsible for in the future. You are then left with the problem of proving it was someone else who used your name and identity to enter into those financial transactions. Your credit could be ruined for many years to come.

Unfortunately, you may not find out about it until legal authorities or credit card collection companies come after you, which can be a very unpleasant experience. You may not even know that your identity has been compromised until you try to purchase a new car or home and the routine credit check reveals the fact that you already own too many cars or too much real estate. Most often, you won't be allowed to buy the car or property until you get the problem cleared up.

The process of rebuilding your identity and credit can be long and tedious. In some cases it may take 10 years or more to iron out all of the wrinkles that have developed.

DON'T BECOME A VICTIM

Since having to deal with the results of identity theft is such an unpleasant process, the best thing is to safeguard yourself against it before it can happen.

Invest in a fireproof file cabinet or safe and store your important personal documents there. If you'd rather not make such a purchase or prefer not to have a safe in your home, you can rent a safe-deposit box at your bank and use the bank's vault as your security box.

Buy a shredder and use it on any bills, credit card offers and other paperwork that contain your name, bank name, credit card or billing information before you throw them away. That will prevent others from getting your financial and personal information by sifting through your trash.

Make sure your credit card number does not appear in its entirety on any credit receipt. It is now against the law for businesses to show the entire number on their receipts. This keeps someone from getting a copy of the receipt and your number. Be aware, though, that some small merchants still use the old "knuckle busters," in which a sliding device is drawn across the credit slip and the card by hand, resulting in an imprint of the complete number, so you must be sure it will be destroyed after the vendor has relayed your information to the credit card company by computer or telephone.

Be careful in situations in which your credit card is carried out of your sight for processing. This can happen in restaurants and some stores. In one Florida restaurant, a waiter swiped hundreds of credit cards into a special hand-held machine and sold the numbers to criminals. If you do not feel comfortable seeing your credit card disappear for some time, ask to go to the cashier with the waiter or salesman. Tell them you had a bad experience and don't let your card out of your sight. More than likely, they will be happy to accommodate you.

Check your credit report at least once a year so that unauthorized charges cannot build up without your knowledge.

Sign up with one of the private companies or credit bureaus that offer insurance and protection services. Make sure you're getting what you want, as these services provide different types of coverage. Some will offer insurance against losses. Others will offer help in putting your credit back together. Some will offer notification regarding inquiries that have been made against your credit, in case it was not you applying for the credit.

Your credit card companies may offer some or all of these services as well. Nowadays, many card companies will call you to verify certain transactions that seem out of the ordinary. For example, if you take a trip and use your credit card in a state other than where you live, you may receive a call from the company about those charges. They are protecting you and themselves against possible fraud.

LIMIT ACCESS TO YOUR PERSONAL INFORMATION

But strangers and thieves aren't the only ones you must guard against. A lot of identity theft occurs when people you know have access to your accounts, credit cards, social security number and driver's license.

Wealthy people who hire assistants, accountants and other financial consultants to help manage their monetary and personal records are always in danger. In some cases, criminals will try to bribe secretaries or assistants for information on their employers. At times, employees who don't feel that they make enough money or are angry at their bosses will steal information and sell it to criminals. It is unpleasant to think such things could happen, but they do.

Patients in hospitals or nursing homes or people being taken care of at home are another group in danger of having their identity stolen. Janitors, orderlies or other healthcare workers have been known to go through the belongings of patients who are medicated or asleep. They will either steal personal items, including jewelry, cash and mementos, or make copies of documents that can be used to steal their identity. Friends and family members need to take precautionary measures and make sure identification, credit cards, checks and other personal papers are locked up in a safe or removed from the room.

Another potentially vulnerable category is people with ex-spouses or former boyfriends or girlfriends who had (or still have) access to their identification and credit cards. There have been cases in which people angry about the separation misused credit cards or sold identity information to get even or realize monetary gain. If you find yourself in circumstances where this could become a problem, the best thing to do is cancel all credit cards and have new ones issued to you as soon as possible. Make sure that the bank removes any authorized co-signers you no longer trust to have your best interests at heart.

DOCUMENT SAFETY ON THE INTERNET

You probably already know that if your computer has a wireless or modem hookup, once you turn it on, you're linked to the whole world. Surf the Internet and you open the door to the information highway. You have almost instant access to places you've never been, places you want to see, and people who may be as far away as the other side of the globe.

At the same time, far way people and other places have access to you.

Every time you do something online, it creates a document trail that exists in cyberspace and can be accessed. If you make a purchase or sign up for a newsletter on a website, some database will store that fact. Many websites, from giants like Amazon to smaller e-tailers, will profile your purchases so they can recommend other products you might be interested in either by e-mail or the next time you visit the site.

Large computers can store billions of pieces of data. This means that your identity and a great deal of personal information about you are potentially available to people to use for criminal purposes, including identity theft.

Online shopping

It used to be that many people were reluctant to shop on the Internet because they were concerned that their credit card information would get stolen. But e-commerce has become as routine as putting on one's shoes in the morning, and millions of people shop online each year. Still, once you give out your credit card or bank account information to make purchases on the Internet, if the website is unsecured, there may be a third party involved during the processing, who has no business knowing any of your financial information.

A simple way to protect yourself is to make sure that any website where you shop uses a secure server. Many online stores already have security built into their shopping systems, promising secure checkouts and purchases. There should be visible notification of this on the checkout page. All valid sites will tell you if the information you're sending is encrypted or if it's going through an open source. If you are not comfortable with the payment process, do not use your credit card to purchase from that site.

After you have made an online purchase, check the charge on your credit card or bank card statement as soon as possible. Make sure that it is the amount you expected and that there is only one charge. Sometimes, if you hit the "send" button that activates the transaction more than once, either by accident or because you didn't think it went through, you may be charged twice. Review your statement again a day or two later to verify that there are no other charges from the site, which might indicate that someone has acquired your information and is using it improperly.

One of the great benefits of the Internet is that we can get online access to our bank account information at any time. This allows us to identify errors or problems before the monthly statement arrives. I would recommend that anyone who feels comfortable using the Internet should set up this kind of banking access.

PERSONAL RECORDS

These days, a great deal of personal information, from driver's licenses to medical records to college and employment records, is available online. Add to that what you yourself put on social networking sites like Facebook, LinkedIn and Myspace, and you can be certain that much of your identity is permanently in cyberspace.

When you have a car accident and are taken to the hospital by an ambulance, all your vital information—medical records, insurance details, police reports—is sent over the air waves while you're en route. Reports about your accident may be "in the system" before you've even arrived at the emergency room, and end up on the Internet.

If your educational history includes attendance at several different colleges, in every case, the admission process required considerable personal information. For several decades, that information has been stored online. More recently, all of your student records, grades, instructor comments and recommendations have probably been stored online as well. What happens to those records? Who has access to them? Can you be sure that they are securely protected, or whether they will be sent elsewhere without your knowledge?

When a loved one dies, what happens to his or her records? Where are those records being sent? How do you know they can't be used by someone who is up to no good? Is there any type of program placed into the system explaining what has happened to the records of the deceased person?

You may not know that there is a national clearinghouse for all the records of individuals across the United States. How safe are those records? Who determines the proper checks and balances, to make sure someone won't give out those records to someone who uses them for base or criminal purposes?

With social security numbers coding everything from medical files to personal financial accounts, it is all too easy for someone who gets access to one of your files to retrieve the rest.

Many of these document and privacy issues are still unsettled because the technology is so new and always changing. No doubt in time, there will be laws and governmental oversight to insure safety and proper use of all this data.

In the meantime, how do you protect yourself?

COMPUTER HACKERS

Every few months there are stories in the news about computer hackers breaching the firewalls of large companies and organizations and gaining illegal access to the records of thousands of Americans. In some cases they are credit card numbers. In a highly publicized case, a glitch by the U.S. Veterans Administration resulted in hundreds of thousands of veterans' medical records being unsecured and open to view.

There is not much you can do about that as an individual except to be aware. If you hear of your bank being compromised, become proactive and start monitoring the transactions on your credit cards. In some cases, the bank will issue you new cards to prevent any negative fallout from such a security breach.

More immediate is the danger from hackers and cyber-geeks who are out to create havoc. If you have spent any time on the Internet, no doubt you have encountered computer viruses. Some are just a minor nuisance. But others are vicious and destructive. They can erase all of your data files and crash your hard drive. Still other viruses can copy all of your documents on the computer (without your knowledge) and send the information to the person that created the virus.

Computer hackers love the element of surprise and thrive on catching people off guard. They look for simple ways to get into your system. Some of their "bugs" come to you via e-mail with an enticing message, counting on your natural sense of curiosity to open it. Once you've done so, the virus or worm will infect your computer and "eat away" at everything until your system is trashed.

VIRUSES AND WORMS

Install a good anti-virus program on your computer. It's an inexpensive way to protect your personal information and files — some basic programs are downloadable free of charge, but it's worth paying the $30 to $50 a year to get the most up-to-date, state-of-the art protection. Be aware, though, that even the best program can only do so much. Hackers keep coming up with new "cyber critters," and anti-virus programmers often play catch-up to the newest "bug" out there. In the meantime, you're vulnerable and must be on guard. Always police your computer system and stay up-to-date in protecting yourself, your documents and your property.

Be wary of programs that claim your computer is infected and offer to run a free scan. Do not allow any programs to be downloaded without researching them ahead of time. Don't simply agree to install something new because you think you have no other choice. Actually look into the program to see if it's necessary or if it may be a hacker trap.

Once you hit "OK" for downloading, you have opened up the doorway for a multitude of possible problems. Look for encryption security on all programs. Go to your local computer store and pick the associates' brains. Talk to local experts about what you can do to stay safe online. Get as much information as you can to be fully prepared and protected from viruses and hackers.

BACKUP PROGRAMS

Because no anti-virus program is fail-safe, it is crucial to have a good backup system in place, so you can restore your files if your computer has come under attack. There are some very good, inexpensive programs available out there. For around $50 a year, you can download software that will back up all the documents on your personal computer to an Internet storage site every time it is turned on. You can continue with your regular computer work or surf the Web while the program operates in the background without interfering with what you're doing.

You can also back up your files yourself and store them in a location separate from your computer. One of the most popular accessories is an external backup hard drive, which you can store anywhere. The drawback is that you must remember to back up your files on a regular basis. Once or twice a week is probably enough.

If you have a larger business or organization, you may need a more powerful system that can back up all of your files at least once a day. In that case, I recommend hiring an information technology (IT) specialist to set up an appropriate system for you. Large companies often have such an expert on staff.

Password protection

Another good way to safeguard against hackers is to use passwords on your computer, especially for your most critical files, such as financial records. This makes it more difficult for a hacker to access your information. If you don't know how to use password protection on your computer, visit your local computer store to ask questions or hire a computer company to set it up for you.

Websites that require you to have an account with them will also ask you to create user names and passwords in order to protect you against unauthorized use.

When creating a password for your own computer or a website, don't use words that someone else can easily guess—the names of your spouse or children, for example. Create a random mixture of letters instead. Include at least two numbers and capitalize one or two letters in the password. If you do this, even if someone guesses the word but does not get the capital letters right, it will not work.

If you have difficulty remembering all of your different passwords—and many people do—write them down for reference, but make sure you keep them in a safe place, and not somewhere they can be easily located if someone happens to rifle through your papers. Above all, don't keep them on a Post-it note attached to your computer.

WIRELESS NETWORKS

If you have a wireless network in your home or office, make sure you either use encrypted WEP (Wired Equivalent Privacy) or a password to gain access. Alternatively, you can set up your network to allow only the MAC (Media Access Control) address of certain machines to access your network. This will keep someone in another apartment or office in your building, or someone driving down the street searching for an open network, from logging on to yours. Another thing you can do to protect yourself is to make sure that the SSID (service set identifier) name of your network won't be broadcast. This will allow only people who have been set up to use the network to find it.

If you are not computer savvy yourself, be sure to use a reputable company to do the installation for you, or have your high school or college-age children do it for you. They have grown up with computers and the Internet, and are often quite proficient with the new technology.

WHAT YOU NEED TO KNOW

I hope you never experience having your identity stolen and the emotional trauma and drain on your time and energy required to fix the problem, but since it is a part of our high-tech age, you need to understand what your rights and liabilities are in the different circumstances where identity theft can take place. The main thing is to have easy, up-to-date access to your financial and credit information.

The sooner you realize someone else is using your credit card or checking account, the sooner you can reduce your liability. Most credit card companies will remove any charges above $50 made by someone who has stolen your cards and identity. However, your checking account could be totally cleaned out if someone were to get their hands on your checks or debit card.

Report any stolen credit cards, debit cards or checks as soon as possible. This will allow the bank to put a "stop payment" on the checks with numbers you haven't personally used. In addition, the bank or credit card companies can cancel your current cards and issue you new ones. This will help limit your losses and liability.

You may need to file police reports concerning where and when your identity and credit cards were stolen. Your banks will have fraud forms they will want you to fill out. In some cases, they require a separate form for each instance of theft, which can be quite a tedious undertaking.

You should immediately notify the three main credit bureaus, TransUnion, Equifax and Experian, so they can put "fraud alerts" on your credit report. They may require their own fraud forms to be filled out, along with copies of all the police reports and banking fraud reports, in order to clear up your credit rating.

If the person or persons are caught, you may end up testifying in court and take many trips to the police station and lawyer's office.

YOUR LICENSES

Many people today carry professional licenses in addition to their state's driver's license, which can be valuable to criminals who know how to make use of it. You will need to notify your professional associations, as well as your state Department of Motor Vehicles (DMV), that your identity and licenses were stolen. Make sure the agencies are aware that criminals could try to use your license. Then, immediately start the process of having your licenses reissued. Of course, it may be more difficult for you to use your identity, as you may have to prove you are the correct person carrying these IDs.

If your social security card (SSC) was lost, you must notify the proper government agency and request a new card. Be sure to indicate that your card may be in the wrong hands. In addition, make sure all other reports you file with the police, banks and credit card companies include notification that your SSC was stolen.

COPING WITH THE AFTERMATH

Finding yourself in the midst of identity theft can create a lot of stress. You may want to join an identity theft support group in your area with others who are dealing with, or have gone through, the same problems. They will be able to give you comfort, provide support and help you with all of the steps you will have to take in order to get your credit and reputation back.

HELP FROM THE GOVERNMENT

Two U.S. government agencies, the Federal Trade Commission (FTC) and the Federal Communication Commission (FCC), are highly involved with identity theft. You can get a lot of valuable information from the FTC, which is the government's central clearinghouse for identity theft information. Its website is www.consumer.gov/idtheft.

Below is some of the information available from the FTC. I have gone into considerable detail because different types of theft have different reporting requirements.

FRAUDULENT BANK ACCOUNT WITHDRAWALS

Different laws determine your legal remedies based on the type of bank fraud you have suffered. For example, state laws protect you against fraud committed by a thief using paper documents, like stolen or counterfeit checks. But if the thief used an electronic fund transfer, federal law applies. Many transactions may seem to be processed electronically but are still considered "paper" transactions. If you're not sure what type of transaction the thief used to commit the fraud, ask the financial institution that did the processing.

FRAUDULENT ELECTRONIC WITHDRAWALS

The Electronic Fund Transfer Act provides consumer protections for transactions involving an ATM or debit card, or other electronic ways to debit or credit an account. It also limits your liability for unauthorized electronic fund transfers. You have 60 days from the date your bank account statement is sent to you to report in writing any money withdrawn from your account without your permission. This includes instances when your ATM or debit card is "skimmed," which is when a thief captures your account number and PIN without your card having been lost or stolen.

If your ATM or debit card is lost or stolen, report it immediately because the amount you can be held responsible for depends on how quickly you report the loss.

- If you report the loss or theft within two business days of discovery, your losses are limited to $50.

- If you report the loss or theft after two business days, but within 60 days after the unauthorized electronic fund transfer appears on your statement, you could lose up to $500 of what the thief withdraws.

■ If you wait more than 60 days to report the loss or theft, you could lose all the money taken from your account.

Visa and MasterCard voluntarily have agreed to limit consumers' liability for unauthorized use of their debit cards in most instances to $50 per card, no matter how much time has elapsed since the discovery of the loss or theft of the card.

The best way to protect yourself in the event of an error or fraudulent transaction is to call the financial institution and follow up in writing by certified letter, return receipt requested, so you can prove when the institution received your letter. Keep a copy of the letter for your records.

After receiving your notification about an error on your statement, the institution generally has 10 business days to investigate. The institution must tell you the results of its findings within three business days after completion. It then must correct the error within one business day after determining that it occurred. If the institution needs more time, it may take up to 45 days to complete the investigation, but only if the money in dispute is returned to your account and you are notified promptly of the credit. At the conclusion of its inquiry, if no error has been found, the institution may take the money back if it sends you a written explanation.

FRAUDULENT CHECKS
AND OTHER "PAPER" TRANSACTIONS

In general, if an identity thief steals your checks or counterfeits checks from your existing bank account, you should stop payment, close the account and ask your bank to notify Chex Systems, Inc. or the check verification service with which it does business. Thus, retailers can be notified not to accept these checks. While no federal law limits your losses if someone uses your checks with a forged signature, or uses another type of "paper" transaction such as a demand draft, state laws may protect you. Most states hold the bank responsible for losses from such transactions. At the same time, most states require you to take reasonable care of your account. For example, you may be held responsible for the forgery if you fail to notify the bank in a timely manner that one of your checks was lost or stolen. Contact your state banking or consumer protection agency for more information.

Contact major check verification companies directly for the following services.

To request that they notify retailers who use their databases not to accept your checks, call:

- TeleCheck at 1-800-710-9898 or 1-800-927-0188

- Certegy, Inc. (previously Equifax) at 1-800-437-5120

To find out if the identity thief has been passing bad checks in your name, call:

- SCAN at 1-800-262-7771

If your check is rejected by a merchant, it may be because an identity thief is using your Magnetic Information Character Recognition (MICR) code (the numbers at the bottom of checks), your driver's license number, or another of your identification numbers. The merchant who rejects your check should give you its check verification company contact information so you can find out what information the thief is using. If you find the thief is using your MICR code, ask your bank to close your checking account and open a new one. If you discover the thief is using your driver's license number or some other identification number, work with your DMV or other identification issuing agency to get new identification with new numbers. Once you have taken the appropriate steps, your checks should be accepted.

FRAUDULENT NEW ACCOUNTS

If you have trouble opening a new checking account, it may be because an identity thief has been opening accounts in your name. Chex Systems, Inc. produces consumer reports specifically about checking accounts and as a consumer reporting company, is subject to the Fair Credit Reporting Act (FCRA). You can request a free copy of your consumer report by contacting Chex Systems, Inc. If you find inaccurate information on your consumer report, follow the procedures that I outline under "Correcting Fraudulent Information in Credit Reports" on the next page. Contact each of the banks where account inquiries were made, too. This will help ensure that any fraudulently opened accounts are closed.

- Call Chex Systems, Inc. at 1-800-428-9623, visit www.chexhelp.com, or fax to 602-659-2197.

- Write to Chex Systems, Inc. Consumer Relations at 7805 Hudson Road, Suite 100, Woodbury, MN, 55125.

BANKRUPTCY FRAUD

If you believe someone has filed for bankruptcy in your name, write to the U.S. Trustee in the region where the bankruptcy was filed. A list of the U.S. Trustee program's regional offices is available at www.usdoj.gov/ust.

In your letter, describe the situation and provide proof of your identity. The U.S. Trustee will make a criminal referral to law enforcement authorities if you provide appropriate documentation to substantiate your claim. You also may want to file a complaint with the U.S. attorney and the FBI in the city where the bankruptcy was filed. The U.S. Trustee does not provide legal representation, legal advice or referrals to lawyers. This means you may need to hire an attorney to help convince the bankruptcy court the filing is fraudulent. The U.S. Trustee does not provide consumers with copies of court documents. You can get them from the bankruptcy clerk's office for a fee.

CORRECTING FRAUDULENT INFORMATION IN CREDIT REPORTS

The Fair Credit Reporting Act (FCRA) establishes procedures for correcting fraudulent information on your credit report and requires your report to be made available only for certain legitimate business needs.

Under the rules of the FCRA, both the consumer reporting company and the information provider (the business that sent the information to the consumer reporting company, such as a bank or credit card company) are responsible for correcting the fraudulent information in your report. To protect your rights under the law, contact both the consumer reporting company and the information provider.

CONSUMER REPORTING COMPANY OBLIGATIONS

Consumer reporting companies will block fraudulent information from appearing on your credit report if you take the following steps: Send them a copy of an identity theft report and a letter telling them what information is fraudulent. The letter also should state that the information does not relate to any transaction you made or authorized. In addition, provide proof of your identity, including your social security number, name, address and any other personal information requested.

The consumer reporting company has four business days to block the fraudulent information after accepting your identity theft report. It also must tell the information provider it has blocked the information. The consumer reporting company may refuse to block the information or remove the block if, for example, you have not told the truth about your identity theft. If the consumer reporting company removes the block or refuses to place the block, it must let you know.

The blocking process is only one way for identity theft victims to deal with fraudulent information. There's also the "reinvestigation process," which was designed to help all consumers dispute errors or inaccuracies on their credit reports.

INFORMATION PROVIDER OBLIGATIONS

Information providers stop reporting fraudulent information to the consumer reporting companies once you send them an identity theft report and a letter explaining that what they're reporting resulted from identity theft. But you must send the report and letter to the address specified by the information provider. Be aware, though, that if the provider later learns that the information did not result from identity theft, it may continue to send it out again.

If a consumer reporting company tells an information provider that it has blocked fraudulent information in your credit report, the information provider may not continue to report the information to the consumer reporting company. The information provider also may not hire someone to collect the debt related to the fraudulent account, or sell the debt to anyone else who would try to collect it.

FRAUDULENT CREDIT CARD CHARGES

The Fair Credit Billing Act establishes procedures for resolving billing errors on your credit card accounts, including fraudulent charges. The law also limits your liability for unauthorized credit card charges to $50 per card.

To take advantage of the law's consumer protection povisions, you must:

■ Write to the creditor at the address given for "billing inquiries," NOT the address for sending your payments. Include your name, address, account number and a description of the billing error, including the amount and date of the error.

■ Send your letter so it reaches the creditor within 60 days after the first bill containing the error was mailed to you. If an identity thief changed the address on your account and you didn't receive the bill, your dispute letter still must reach the creditor within 60 days of when the creditor would have mailed the bill. This is one reason it's essential to keep track of your billing statements and follow up quickly if your bills don't arrive on time.

■ You should send your letter by certified mail and request a return receipt. It becomes your proof of the date the creditor received the letter. Include copies (NOT originals) of your police report or other documents that support your position. Keep a copy of your dispute letter.

■ The creditor must acknowledge your complaint in writing within 30 days after receiving it, unless the problem has been resolved. The creditor must resolve the dispute within two billing cycles (but not more than 90 days) after receiving your letter.

CRIMINAL VIOLATIONS

Procedures to correct your record within criminal justice databases can vary from state to state and even from county to county. Some states have enacted laws with special procedures for identity theft victims to follow to clear their names. You should check with the office of your state attorney general, but you can use the following information as a general guide.

If wrongful criminal violations are attributed to your name, contact the police or sheriff's department that originally arrested the person using your identity, or the court agency that issued the warrant for the arrest. File an impersonation report with the police or sheriff's department and confirm your identity by asking the police department to take a full set of your fingerprints, photograph you and make copies of your photo identification documents, like your driver's license, passport or travel visa. To establish your innocence, ask the police to compare the prints and photographs with those of the imposter.

If the arrest warrant is from a state or county other than where you live, ask your local police department to send the impersonation report to the police department in the jurisdiction where the arrest warrant, traffic citation or criminal conviction originated.

The law enforcement agency should then recall any warrants and issue a "clearance letter" or "certificate of release" (if you were arrested or booked). You'll need to keep this document with you at all times in case you're wrongly arrested again. Ask the law enforcement agency to file the record of the follow-up investigation establishing your innocence with the district attorney (D.A.) and/ or court where the crime took place. This will result in an amended complaint. Once your name is recorded in a criminal database, it's unlikely it will be completely removed from the official record. Ask that the "key name" or "primary name" be changed from your name to the imposter's name (or to "John Doe" if the imposter's true identity is not known), with your name noted as an alias.

You'll also want to clear your name in the court records. To do this, you'll need to determine which state law(s) will help you with this and how. If your state has no formal procedure for clearing your record, contact the D.A.'s office in the county where the case was originally prosecuted. Ask the D.A.'s office for the appropriate court records needed to clear your name. You may have to hire a criminal defense attorney to help with the situation. Contact Legal Services in your state or your local bar association for help in finding an attorney.

Finally, contact your state DMV to find out if your driver's license is being used by the identity thief. Ask that your files be flagged for possible fraud.

DEBT COLLECTORS

The Fair Debt Collection Practices Act prohibits debt collectors from using unfair or deceptive practices to collect overdue bills a creditor has forwarded for collection, even if those bills don't result from identity theft. You can stop a debt collector from contacting you in the following ways:

- Write a letter immediately to the collection agency telling it to stop. Once the debt collector receives your letter, the company may not contact you again with two exceptions: It may tell you there will be no further contact, and it may tell you that the debt collector or the creditor intends to take some specific action.

- Send a letter to the collection agency within 30 days of receiving written notice of the debt, telling it you do not owe the money. Include copies of documents that support your position. Appending a copy (NOT original) of your police report may be useful. In that case, a collector can renew collection activities only if it sends you proof of the debt.

- If you don't have documentation to support your position, be as specific as possible about why the debt collector is mistaken. The debt collector is responsible for sending you proof that you're wrong. For example, if the debt you're disputing originates from a credit card you never applied for, ask for a copy of the application with the applicant's signature. Then, you can prove it's not your signature.

- If you tell the debt collector you are a victim of identity theft and it is collecting the debt for another company, the debt collector must tell the company you may be a victim of identity theft.

- While you can stop a debt collector from contacting you, it won't get rid of the debt itself. It's important to contact the company that originally opened the account to dispute the debt, otherwise the company may send it to a different debt collector, report it on your credit report or initiate a lawsuit to collect on the debt.

FALSE DRIVER'S LICENSE

If you think your name or social security number is being used by an identity thief to get a driver's license or a non-driver's ID card, contact your state DMV. If the DMV uses your social security number as your driver's license number, ask to substitute another number.

INVESTMENT FRAUD

The U.S. Securities and Exchange Commission's (SEC) Office of Investor Education and Assistance serves investors who complain to the SEC about investment fraud or the mishandling of their investments by securities professionals. If you believe an identity thief has tampered with your securities investments or a brokerage account, immediately report it to your broker or account manager and to the SEC.

You can file a complaint with the SEC's Complaint Center at www.sec.gov/complaint.shtml. Include as much detail as possible. If you don't have Internet access, write to the SEC Office of

Investor Education and Assistance, 450 Fifth Street, N.W., Washington, D.C., 20549-0213. For answers to general questions, call 202-942-7040.

MAIL THEFT

The U.S. Postal Inspection Service (USPIS) is the law enforcement arm of the U.S. Postal Service and investigates cases of identity theft. The USPIS has primary jurisdiction in all matters infringing on the integrity of the U.S. mail. If an identity thief has stolen your mail to get new credit cards, bank or credit card statements, prescreened credit offers, or tax information, or has falsified change-of-address forms or obtained your personal information through a fraud conducted by mail, report it to your local postal inspector.

You can locate the USPIS district office nearest you by calling your local post office or by visiting www.postalinspectors.uspis.gov.

PASSPORT FRAUD

If you've lost your passport or believe it was stolen or is being used fraudulently, contact the United States Department of State (USDS) through www.travel.state.gov/passport/passport_1738.html or call 1-800-877-8339 to locate a local USDS field office.

PHONE FRAUD

If an identity thief has established phone service in your name, is making unauthorized calls that seem to come from and are billed to your cellular phone, or is using your calling card and PIN, contact your service provider immediately to cancel the account and/or calling card. Open new accounts and choose new PINs. If you're having trouble getting fraudulent phone charges removed from your account or getting an unauthorized account closed, contact the appropriate agency below.

- For local service, contact your state Public Utility Commission.

- For cellular phones and long distance, contact the Federal Communications Commission (FCC) at www.fcc.gov. The FCC regulates interstate and international communications by radio, television, wire, satellite and cable. Call 1-888-CALL-FCC or TTY: 1-888-TELL-FCC. Write to the Federal Communications Commission, Consumer Information Bureau at 445 12th Street, S.W., Room 5A863, Washington, D.C., 20554. You can file complaints online at www. fcc.gov or e-mail your questions to fccinfo@fcc.gov.

SOCIAL SECURITY NUMBER MISUSE

If you have specific information regarding social security number misuse, which involves the buying or selling of social security cards, may be related to terrorist activity, or is designed to obtain social security benefits, contact the Social Security Administration (SSA) Office of the Inspector General. You may file a complaint online at www.socialsecurity.gov/oig, call 1-800-269-0271, fax to 410-597-0118, or write to the SSA Fraud Hotline, P.O. Box 17768, Baltimore, MD, 21235.

You also may call SSA at 1-800-772-1213 to verify the accuracy of the earnings reported on your social security number, request a copy of your social security statement or get a replacement social security card if yours is lost or stolen. Follow up in writing.

STUDENT LOAN FRAUD

If someone gets access to your personal information and takes out a student loan in your name, as soon as you become aware of it contact the school or program that opened the student loan and close it. At the same time, report the fraudulent loan to the U.S. Department of Education.

■ Call the Inspector General's hotline at 1-800-MIS-USED.

■ Visit www.ed.gov/about/offices/list/oig/ hot-line.html?src=rt.

■ Write to the Office of Inspector General, U.S. Department of Education, 400 Maryland Avenue, S.W., Washington, D.C., 20202-1510.

Tax fraud

The Internal Revenue Service (IRS) is responsible for administering and enforcing tax laws. Identity fraud may occur as it relates directly to your tax records. Visit www.irs.gov and type in the key words "Identity Theft" for more information.

If you have an unresolved issue related to identity theft, or you have suffered or are about to suffer a significant hardship as a result of the administration of the tax laws, visit the IRS Taxpayer Advocate Service at www.irs.gov/advocate/ or call 1-877-777-4778.

If you suspect or know of an individual or company who is not complying with the tax law, report it to the Internal Revenue Service criminal investigation informant hotline by calling 1-800-829-0433 or visiting www.irs.gov and typing in the key words "Tax Fraud."

What if I still have a problem?

There are cases in which victims do everything right and still spend years dealing with problems related to identity theft. The good news is that most victims can get their cases resolved by being vigilant, assertive and organized. Don't procrastinate on contacting companies to address the problems. Don't be afraid to go up the chain of command or make complaints, if necessary. Keep organized files. If you haven't filed a complaint with the FTC or updated it, you should do so and provide details of the problems that you are having.

You also can call the hotline 1-877-ID-THEFT to talk with one of its counselors. If your problems are stemming from the failure of a party to perform its legal obligations, you may want to consult an attorney. You can contact Legal Services in your state or your local bar association for help in finding an attorney who specializes in such violations.

CONCLUSION

It may take a great deal of time and effort on your part to restore your life to normal after you've been a victim of identity theft, but the good news is that you can do it. It may demand persistence, determination and the patience of a saint—especially when dealing with mind-numbing requirements of some bureaucracies—but the effort to reclaim your life and your good name is worth it.

5-POINT PLAN

1.   Make sure your credit card receipts only reveal the last four digits.

2.   Keep your most important personal records in a safe at home or a safe-deposit box at a bank.

3.   Invest in a shredder and run all your personal documents through it before you throw them out.

4.   Make sure your computer files are password protected.

5.   Invest in anti-virus and backup software for your computer.

EPILOGUE

If you have come this far, I want to congratulate you both for your interest and persistence. The fact that you took the time and effort not only speaks to your commitment to safety for you and your family, but virtually guarantees that you will be better prepared than most to deal with the challenges life in the United States presents nowadays.

I believe that fundamentally most people are good and want the best for themselves and their family, friends, neighbors and fellow citizens. It is only a relatively small minority of criminals that attempts to use shortcuts to obtain money and material things the rest of us work for diligently. We should not allow them to diminish our quality of life, and if you follow the safety precautions I have outlined in this book, they won't be able to.

I also believe that individuals have more power and ability to help themselves than they might think. When we're confronted by nightly news accounts of criminal acts, we can get a skewed sense of reality. So it is important to both keep a good perspective and prepare ourselves for worst-case-scenarios without descending into excessive worry and fear. You can do much more than you think to make a difference

Once again, the more aware we become of our environment, both as individuals and larger groups within our society, the more likely we are to come up with solutions that will allow us to enjoy life to the fullest without falling victim to predators that want to deprive us of our rights and freedom.

We live in a great country, and together we can ensure that we will live here in relative harmony and without fear, ready to pursue the American Dream and make a better future for ourselves and our children.

I would be happy to hear from you and welcome your thoughts, stories and suggestions on further safety measures that can help us all live the lives we want to. You can contact me at my specific e-mail address: r.daniels@theultimatelock.com.

Ron Daniels

APPENDIX

THE ULTIMATE LOCK

I have recommended a number of times in this book that the best way to secure your home and protect yourself and your family is to install high-security locks on the entrance doors to your house, as well as on the door to an interior "safe room."

I believe this so strongly that I have taken the time to design such a security lock myself with the assistance of NASA's Space Alliance Technology Outreach Program (SATOP). I call it The Ultimate Lock, and I can guarantee that it will perform at the highest level to ensure safety in your home. You can find out more about it at www.theultimatelock.com.

The Ultimate Lock was featured on national television on the Montel Williams Show and has been awarded contracts through municipalities and FEMA.

The lock will withstand up to 4,000 pounds of pressure, and has held up successfully in tests involving 40-pound and 70-pound police battering rams. It works in conjunction with ordinary deadbolt locks, so that a stranger won't be aware that it is there. The first time a criminal tries to kick in the door, it will feel like he's hitting a brick wall, and the intense pain from the shock of the impact will make him think twice about trying it again. Any other attempts on his part will meet with the same result, and he is likely to give up and go away.

Another important feature of The Ultimate Lock is a safety lock-out feature. This allows you to prevent anyone from coming into your home with just the push of a button. Once the lock-out feature is on, it renders any key useless. Even family members who

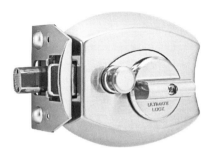

have keys to the house won't be able to get in once you have engaged the lock-out function. You are in full control.

The Ultimate Lock fits any door and can turn a bedroom, bathroom, or even the basement into a safe room (so long as the door is solid wood or metal).

In my view—and I'm not just saying this because I created it—The Ultimate Lock is the best protective device available today for securing your home and providing safety for you and your family.

INDEX

RON DANIELS

A native of Houston, Texas, Ron Daniels holds both Bachelor and Master of Science degrees in criminal justice management. After graduating with honors from the University of Houston Law Enforcement Academy, he served as public relations officer and oversaw both the D.A.R.E. (Drug Abuse Resistance Education) and G.R.E.A.T. (Gang Resistance Education and Training) programs for Harris County Constable Precinct 7. Formally trained in advanced dignitary (VIP) protection, Daniels also holds a Master Peace Officer Certification, the highest accreditation possible for a police officer. Prior to his career in law enforcement, Daniels launched a number of successful business ventures. Currently president and CEO of Millennium Lock, Inc., and the inventor of The Ultimate Lock, he has made it a mission in his life to help people become safe and secure. He lives with his wife, Sheila, and their four children in Sugar Land, Texas.